# HUMORS AND SUBSTANCES

## *Ideas of the Body in New Guinea*

PAMELA J. STEWART AND ANDREW STRATHERN

With contributions by Ien Courtens and Dianne van Oosterhout

BERGIN & GARVEY
Westport, Connecticut • London

**Library of Congress Cataloging-in-Publication Data**

Stewart, Pamela J.
Humors and substances : ideas of the body in New Guinea / written and edited by Pamela J. Stewart and Andrew Strathern.
p. cm.
Includes bibliographical references and index.
ISBN 0–89789–762–5 (alk. paper)
1. Ethnology—New Guinea. 2. Body, Human—Social aspects—New Guinea. 3. Body fluids—Social aspects—New Guinea. 4. Rites and ceremonies—New Guinea. 5. New Guinea—Social life and customs. I. Title: Ideas of the body in New Guinea. II. Strathern, Andrew. III. Title.
GN671.N5S86 2001
306.4—dc21 00–031204

British Library Cataloguing in Publication Data is available.



Library of Congress Catalog Card Number: 00–031204
ISBN: 0–89789–762–5

First published in 2001

Bergin & Garvey, 88 Post Road West, Westport, CT 06881
An imprint of Greenwood Publishing Group, Inc.
www.greenwood.com

Printed in the United States of America

The paper used in this book complies with the Permanent Paper Standard issued by the National Information Standards Organization (Z39.48–1984).

10 9 8 7 6 5 4 3 2 1

**Copyright Acknowledgments**

The authors and the publisher gratefully acknowledge permission for use of the following material:

Extracts from Pamela J. Stewart and Andrew Strathern, "Politics and poetics mirrored in indigenous stone objects," *Journal of the Polynesian Society* 108 (1): 69–90. Reprinted with permission.

Extracts from Pamela J. Stewart and Andrew Strathern, "Body and mind in Mount Hagen, Highlands Papua New Guinea," *Anthropology of Consciousness*, forthcoming.

# Contents

# Preface

Writings about the human body as a focus of anthropological analysis have proliferated greatly since 1990. Broadly speaking, these writings have tended to revolve around two themes. One approach has been to see the body as a register of cultural values and social forces. In counterpoint, others have stressed the experiential and active role of the body in shaping personal senses of agency. In the first approach, the body is seen as passive, in the second as active. The relationship between mind and body runs across the two themes. In both approaches, the body is in fact seen as an aspect of the whole person, and therefore includes elements of the mind: an idea that is expressed in the term "embodiment."

The special contribution that can be made to these thematic concerns from the perspective of cross-cultural ethnography is that a comparative approach enables us to understand how concepts of the body itself vary, and therefore variably intersect with issues of symbolism, agency, and practice. In turn, an important dimension of such concepts has to do with the ways in which the vital, living sources of being within the body are perceived. The category "humors and substances" is designed to target this dimension. Humoral ideas have been found to be significant in several parts of the world, including Europe, Latin America, and Asia. They did not, however, enter significantly into discussions about ideas of the person in the anthropology of New Guinea until the 1990s, and although there have been references to this theme in the literature, the topic remains a valuable one for careful cross-cultural exploration. This book makes a distinctive contribution to that end, in a number of ways.

First, to the idea of embodiment we add the concept of the cosmos. Not only is the human body realized and expressed as a reality in cultural terms, and culture also in bodily terms, but cultural ideas in general are set into overarching notions of a world beyond each individual person to which the body belongs. In New Guinea this cosmos is not to be seen as an eternal, unchanging, hierarchical entity. It is a world of flow and change encompassing the whole environment as experienced and perceived by people, and the body is a constituent part of these processes of change, just as the soul or spirit is. At birth, the body's part in the cosmos is definitively revealed, and at death its process of alteration and transformation back into the cosmos at large is set into motion. The dynamic relationship of encompassment and participation between the body and the cosmos explains why the body becomes a part of a universe of signs and why these signs are deeply involved in processes of change. For the Duna and Huli people, for example, in the Southern Highlands of Papua New Guinea, the contemporary condition of people's bodies is taken as a sign of a cosmic decline and a moral deterioration in society that needs to be addressed and corrected. Premature bodily maturation and early rather than delayed entry into sexual activity are taken as markers of an overall historical speeding up and compression of time and generations that mark a point of potential major change in the cosmos at large.

Second, this mutual implication of body, cosmos, and historical change provides the overall setting within which notions of agency and sociality are played out. Persons express agency, both as parts of the cosmos and in terms of their social networks. Sociality itself is a part of a wider set of cosmic processes. Individual creativity, innovation, and resistance to social power are all expressed through concepts that correspond to ideas of mind that exist in a symbiotic and dialectical relationship with ideas of the body. For the Hagen people of the Western Highlands Province of Papua New Guinea, mind, or *noman*, is in a certain sense a distinguishing characteristic of people as compared with other creatures; yet in another sense everything has its *noman*, its customary disposition to behave and react in certain ways. What distinguishes humans is their capacity to think and choose, and therefore to be conscious partners in the management of the cosmos.

Third, the concepts of the cosmos and of humors and substances, when taken together, assist greatly in mediating ideas of mind/body distinctiveness. While mind and soul are in some ways seen as distinct from the body, this does not necessarily mean that they are thought of in the abstract, as on different planes of being from the body. In discussions of this sort it is important to look at indigenous concepts. In this regard detailed ethnography has an important part to play. Our discussion in Chapter 7 of the idea of "mind substance" as a translation for *noman* nicely illustrates this point. When set into an overall picture of flows of substance in the body, it becomes clear that the *noman* is seen as linked to *peng konya*, head substance, and this in turn to grease/body fat (*kopong*) and reproductive fluids generally. Any absolute antinomy between *noman* and body is thus broken down, even though Hageners also say that the *noman* is not like the organs of the body such as the heart, lungs, and liver, and cannot be seen if the body is cut open. It is clearly an emergent expression of the fact of consciousness, and Hageners wish both to separate this in some sense from the physical organs of the body and at the same time to link it to vital bodily processes that integrate the body itself into the cosmos.

As we explain in Chapter 1, we make a composite category of humors and substances generally, while singling out humors as the most important or significant constituents in the overall flow of life. To some extent this is a subjective evaluation, but its purpose is comparative, since it enables us to make cross-cultural explorations of ideas about, for example, "blood" or "grease/body fat." One of our aims in this volume is also commensurate with the outlines in our earlier volume, *The Python's Back: Pathways of Comparison Between Indonesia and Melanesia* (Strathern and Stewart 2000). That is, the concept of humors facilitates the bringing together of ideas about the body beyond the artificial confines of Papua New Guinea as an arena for ethnographic comparison-making. This is because humoral ideas of one kind or another are found widely in Southeast Asia, with meanings and functions entirely analogous to those in Papua New Guinea. The geopolitical space of Irian Jaya forms in this context a useful bridge between Melanesia, including Papua New Guinea, and Indonesia or Malaysia. For this reason we are pleased to be able to include in the present volume two firsthand studies from Irian Jaya, one by Ien Courtens and the other by Dianne van Oosterhout, both of which aptly show that a focus on the body, and on humors and substances, provides an excellent platform for discerning cross-cultural similarities of themes. These themes relate to a host of domains in ethnographic analysis: social structure, gender, witchcraft, history of contact with "outsiders," notions about food, ancestors, sacrifice, and reciprocity in general. In brief, the body, as perceived culturally in terms of humors and substances, itself becomes a vehicle for cross-cultural comparison-making, one that integrates otherwise separable themes around a single focus.

Finally, here this focus on the body also gives us a novel mode of entry into the discussion of social change. The concept, as we use it, is thus not a timeless constant, but one that encompasses historical variability, and is in fact a vehicle for sensitive indications of change, at least in the context of New Guinea. The reason is, as we have noted above, that the body and the cosmos are linked in both moral and physical terms, and the realm of the physical is informed by ideas of morality, ancestrality, force, and flows of power. This question of the body and change is one that is bound to gain urgency with the advance of new epidemics such as AIDS. New categorizations of disease conditions are likely to emerge that build on, rather than negate, old humoral ideas. For example, in a February 2000 communication from a collaborator in the Hagen area we learned that two middle-aged men of his clan had untowardly died on the second day of the new millennium, January 2, 2000. He reported that "the doctors" had told them that one of these men had "blood cancer." While this description might relate to a biomedically diagnosed condition, in his representation it also relates to ideas about blood and life force, or may also be an inchoate way of signaling other causes of the death. It is imperative to have a good understanding of the local ideas out of which new transcultural notions of a hybrid kind are developing. This book also represents a step in the direction of meeting that need and should provide materials for further comparative analysis with studies from other geographical areas.

## REFERENCE

Strathern, Andrew, and Pamela J. Stewart. 2000. *The Python's Back: Pathways of Comparison Between Indonesia and Melanesia.* Westport, CT: Bergin and Garvey.

# Acknowledgments

We wish to thank the people of Papua New Guinea with whom we have worked and the relevant government organizations for granting research permits. In this work some abbreviations and/or pseudonyms may have been used where appropriate. We have paraphrased some translations slightly for clarity of exposition where necessary. Special thanks also go to our contributors, Ien Courtens and Dianne van Oosterhout, for their Chapters on Irian Jaya, now called West Papua.

We wish to thank the National Museum of Ethnology in Osaka, Japan for providing us with work space and positions as visiting Researcher and Visiting Scholar during April, May, and June of 2000 when we were working on the copyedited text of this manuscript.

We want to thank the Press for their continued interest in publishing scholarly works such as this book. Special thanks go to Jane Garry who was enthusiastic and supportive of our project from the onset. Thanks also go to the production staff, especially Linda Ellis-Stiewing.

# CHAPTER 1

# Introduction: Gathering the Threads of the Flow of Life

*Pamela J. Stewart and Andrew Strathern*

Notions of bodily fluids and the importance of these substances are part of every human's daily concerns. Heightened awareness about the transmission of sexual fluids in an age where sexually transmitted diseases are a notable concern is just one aspect of how we perceive our bodily fluids and the exchange of those substances with others. Many new concerns are in the minds of people today over genetically engineered human products such as hormones for treatment of disease states. Also, moral, ethical, and psychological concerns about reproductive technologies have entered into the mix of humanist concerns about the future of our species. A better understanding of how people think about their bodies and the substances that constitute them should facilitate the conceptualization of developing arenas in which substances are transferred and transformed in new and unfamiliar ways, and the clarification of how this process impacts our self-images and our relationships with others.

The geographic focus of this book is New Guinea, and one of our aims is to stress how in this part of the world the substances of human bodies define and delineate social relations, and are in turn given worth and significance through those relationships. Ideas of humors and bodily substances run through the mythology, folklore, ritual, and everyday practices of many of the peoples of New Guinea and the wider Pacific region, like so many threads connecting the themes of custom, social structure, life history, and the world of imagination. A good deal has been written about ideas of the body in general in these New Guinea cultures (see map 1), both in passing within the contexts of other frameworks of writing and more specifically in tune with the anthropological interest in embodiment theory (including the recognition of the body as a receptor of stimuli that are transmitted and processed into mental and physical responses) (see, e.g., Csordas 1994). Within these writings we can discern a particular emphasis on discrete substances as the carriers and extensions of important aspects of persons as social actors: blood, reproductive fluids, fat (grease), water, bones, sweat, and excreta, for example, all figure prominently in people's discussions of how they conceptualize social relationships.

These parts and emanations of the person both constitute the actual physical makeup and the internal states of persons and also can function as transmissible and transposable signs of persons in exchange with one another. They stand both for what is intimate, particular, and hidden, and for what is social, general, and revealed in interactions. In this book we pull together several of the ethnographic themes that stem from this basic point, seeing our enterprise as one of pursuing threads of practice across cultural contexts and of gathering these threads together in a synoptic fashion. The perspectives we offer are well established in existing literature, but our aim is to highlight the theme of humors and substances, and give it a central place in understanding the contexts we discuss.

Humoral systems have been discussed quite extensively in anthropological literature, mostly for the ancient Greek and contemporary Mediterranean areas, Latin America, and Asia (e.g., Lloyd 1973; Foster 1994; Zimmerman 1982). More recently there has been an attempt to extend the concept of humors into the ethnography of New Guinea and the Pacific (Strathern 1996; Strathern and Stewart 1999a). The point of doing so is to extrapolate from the other areas elements of definition that are applicable to the New Guinea contexts. In the ancient Greek system we see the following combination of ideas: (1) a view that the world and the human body derive from fundamental elements such as fire, water, air, and earth; (2) a view that the human body contains humors such as bile (yellow or black), blood, and phlegm, which influence situational behavioral patterns or character; (3) a view that for health, these elements should be in balance, and that the balance is affected seasonally by food intake (e.g., causing a relatively wet or dry state) and by emotional states; and (4) a view that the body, foods, and other elements may be in a hot, cold, or cool condition, and that a balance between hot and cold is required for health.

Of these "classic" elements, the ones we find most clearly in New Guinea are 2 (i.e., bodily fluids modify behavior) and 4 (i.e., bodily thermal states alter health), although traces of the others also appear. The humoral picture of the body is, in New Guinea, closely intertwined with ideas about sexual activity, maturation, and gender relations, and is applied in contemporary contexts to circumstances of social change. Health and sickness, fertility and decay, female and male characteristics, may all be expressed in terms of notions of particular

**Map 1**
**The Island of New Guinea**

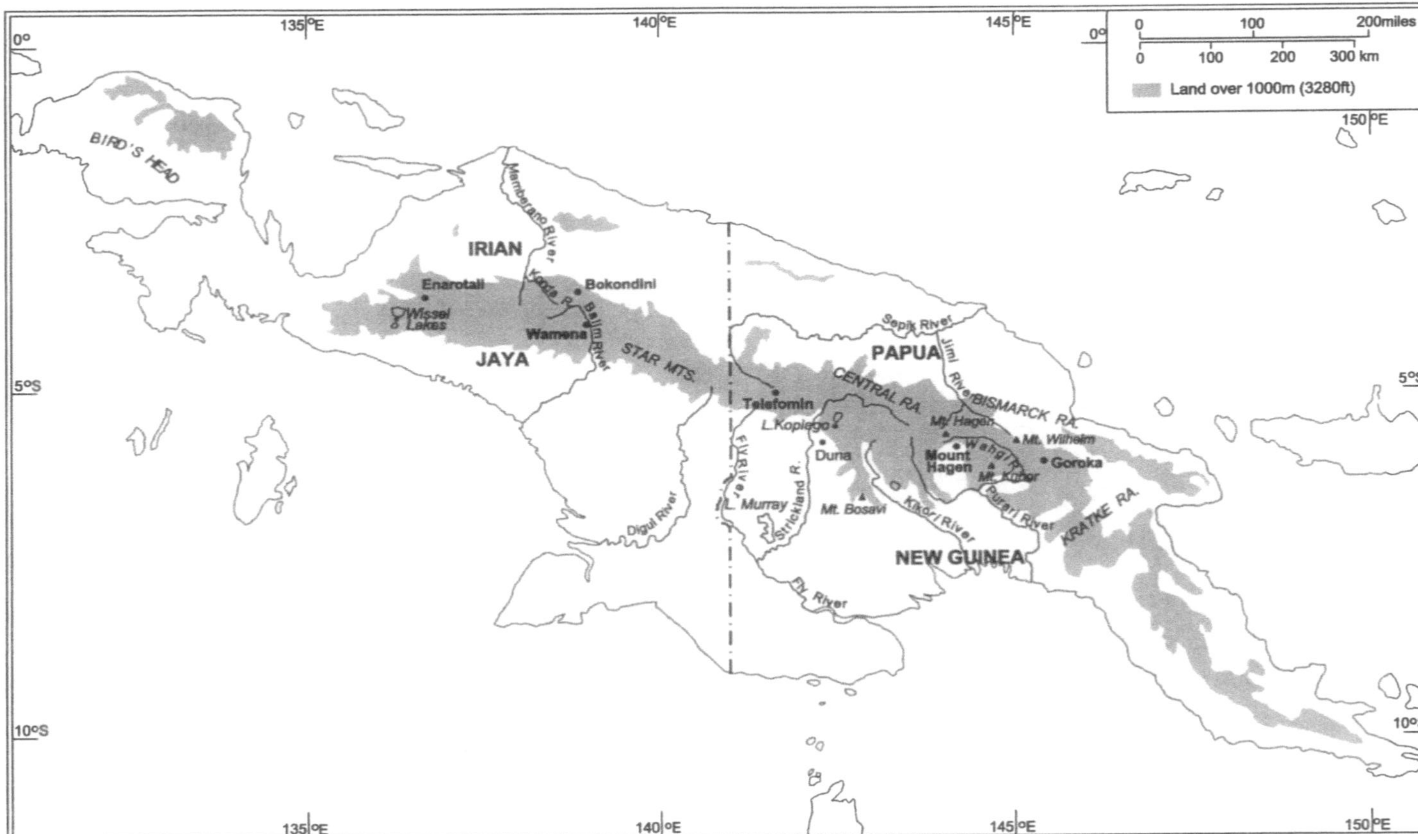

humors, such as blood and grease/water, and by way of expressions having to do with the dimensions of the hot and the cold, or the wet and the dry.

To take two examples well established in the literature: (1) Anna Meigs has described, for the Hua of the Eastern Highlands of Papua New Guinea, how males are associated with things that are hard and dry and females with the soft and the wet, but each sex has to maintain a bodily balance between these qualities by adjusting their intake of foods (Meigs 1984); (2) Jeffrey Clark reports for the Huli of the Southern Highlands Province that ideas of sexuality revolved around blood and its condition, which affected "beauty" for both sexes. Unregulated sexual behavior was thought to deplete men's semen and also to "finish" women's blood through pregnancy. Women's vaginas were said to be "hot," and therefore potentially dangerous for men. Semen was thought to be cooling, and the combination of fluids in sexual intercourse resulted in a harmonious balance. Contemporary prostitutes, whose uncontrolled behavior is said to threaten the reproductive order of the world, are said to have vaginas not only "like fire" but also "like coffee," a commodity sold for money. Social change and immorality are associated with inordinate heat that is inimical to balance and fertility. Bachelors' rites among the Huli centered at least partly on the symbolism of cool, life-giving water, and were called *iba giya* (water-giving) (Clark 1997:198–202). The parallels in this last regard with Hagen in the Highlands of Papua New Guinea will be made clear in Chapter 6. There appears to be some overlap between water and semen here, but water is the more encompassing cosmic element. We can regard both water and semen, as well as breast milk, as "humors" of the body, or we can consider them as "substances." As we explain below, for our purposes here we wish to make a specific distinction between these two terms.

Why the two terms, humors and substances? By humors we refer to elements such as blood, water, fat, and reproductive fluids that are seen by people as important constituents of the physical and moral constitution of persons, sometimes defining their self-worth and acceptance by their social peers. As is the case with emotions, ideas about such elements tend to form limited sets and to constitute a core of notions on which concepts of personhood are built. We can speak of "two humor" or "three humor" cases in this way, referring to the fact that blood and grease/fat are the two most significant elements in some instances, whereas in others, three elements such as blood, fat, and water may be involved (Strathern and Stewart 1999a). These limited or core sets of notions are in turn embedded in a wider universe of ideas that we call substances. We use this term broadly to include elements such as bone, which can be a highly significant, enduring aspect of the person, and therefore comes to stand for notions of continuity and accession to power beyond death. We also include whatever physical elements people themselves may emphasize as significant in certain contexts, for example saliva, spittle, or sweat, and body parts like hair, skin, nails, and other tissues. All of these substances are elements of communication that send signals outward from one entity to another person, many people, and the environment, either directly or through objects which carry the message of the sender (e.g., gifts and exchange valuables). They are also items that can be used by enemies to make sorcery against the body of the person who has discharged those substances (Stewart and Strathern 1997, 1999c). Speech also is, of course, an important aspect of communication, but in this book we devote our main attention to the flow of nonverbal communicative substances.

What we are talking about by way of humors and substances are the communicative ontological signals that are transmitted through the framework of perceptions that the receiver imposes upon them. The machinery involved here encompasses the five senses (sight, smell, touch, hearing, and taste) at the phenomenological level as well as the cultural imprints and neural networks that constitute "mind." We devote an entire chapter to the concept of *noman* (i.e., mind, will, agency, intention, sensibility, consciousness) in the Hagen area of the Western Highlands Province of Papua New Guinea) as an exercise to understand better the logic that the Hageners employ in their translation and transformation of sensory stimuli and their reflections on these stimuli.

In our usage, then, humors are a special subset of substances in general, so our term "humors and substances" has to be seen as meaning "humors and substances in general." Given the distinction, we do not mean to use it in a rigidly typological way, but as a background device of description where appropriate. We also do not intend the idea of humors and substances to encompass everything that can be said about the person. The chapter that we devote to the detailed consideration of a set of ideas about mind in the Hagen area demonstrates that the *noman* for the Hageners is linked to and in constant interplay with other aspects of the person, including, for example, "blood" and "grease" (fat, semen, breast milk), and yet is not subsumed within these as an immanent part of them. There is therefore a kind of duality in their thought, but it is not the duality of a mind/body split; rather, it is an image of interplay and mutual influence closer to contemporary understandings of mind and body in general (see Damasio 1999).

Consideration of this point can lead us to ask in general how people's ideas of extensions of the person work, whether through concepts of material forces carried in humors and substances, and in wealth items or food, or through notions of projections of "mental substances" or what can be called agency. The actual situation, we suggest, lies in between the material and the immaterial. Emanations of the person consist equally of the transmission of substances and of effects of agency (i.e., the transmission of "mental substances"), such as are seen in physical acts and social acts of speaking, giving, withholding, threatening, appeasing, and the like, all of which by nature have an embodied dimension of the physicality of the human organism. What in English usage we refer to as the disembodied realm of mind or spirit is seen by many New Guinea peoples as another realm of being, physical in aspect but not so readily apprehended, and clearly challenged and altered by the entrapment of the body. Spirits continue to perform actions that are analogous to those of living people, as in this passage by the Papuan novelist Vincent Eri, from Moveave village in the Gulf Province of Papua New Guinea, writing of proper forms of cooking:

> The family should not be exposed to the dangers of eating food that was prepared before the eyes of many people. Their eyes ate the food as it was being cooked. And you never know: spirits of the dead, wandering by the pot of food, might spit into it. (Eri 1976:19)

Here, two vivid physicalities are involved: human eyes eat and spirit mouths spit, in each case expressing the power to influence the world. If eyes can "eat," certainly spirits can "spit." Expressions of this kind create a picture of the world that criss-crosses the boundaries of what we might otherwise call the symbolic/metaphorical and the real/literal.

Another excellent example of this is detailed in the Hagen myth of the spirit beings Ntim and Ntam (Vicedom and Tischner 1943; Strathern 1977b: 123–125).

**The Spirits Ntim and Ntam**

The story tells how two spirit men called Ntim and Ntam saw a young human girl whom they wished to marry but two human men named Towa and Kawokla also wished to marry her. The human men killed pigs and presented them to the girl's parents as brideprice and then took the girl off to their own village. When the spirit men arrived at the girl's parents house they heard of what had happened and killed the parents, destroying their house and gardens in a rage. "One day Towa and Kawokla decided to collect lianas [vine ropes] in the woods, and they took the wife with them, leaving her in a hunting-hut while they went out to hunt. . . . She heard a Rompena bird suddenly beginning to sing: 'Ajamb Waklop, look out, here come the spirits of Ntim and Ntam.' Hearing this, the woman hurried back to her hut. The two spirits did come, and told her to go along with them. She cried, but they insisted, so she pulled out her hair and strewed it around the front of the hut, took her cowrie-necklace and other valuables out of her netbag and went with them. They came to a steep drop on one side of the way. One of the spirits ran off down this and from there he shot the woman with an arrow. They left her body lying there and went away. The woman's spirit went home and cooked a meal in the hunting-hut and the men, who returned with their catch, received their food from her. After the meal, she announced to them: 'Live well, you two men! I have now become the wife of the spirits Ntim and Ntam and am going to see them.'" At this point one of the two human husbands followed the ghost wife until he collapsed in exhaustion. He was found by an old woman to whom he told his story. The man cut off one of his fingers and the old woman mixed the blood that dripped from the finger with food that she took off to feed to the ghost wife. The old woman asked the ghost wife if she would like to see her human husband again. She said yes, very much, but she was now in the land of the dead, so how could it be managed? The old woman brought her husband to her and the two recognized each other and went home to his settlement. Subsequently, the woman bore a son who grew old enough to talk and one day when his mother went to gather sweet potatoes in her garden the boy began to cry and scream, which upset the father who spoke hastily and said "What are you crying for?

You owe your life to me. Your mother was dead and I cut off my finger and gave her my blood and brought her back to life. Do you hear?" When the woman returned from her garden she was so upset at what her husband had revealed that she hanged herself in the night. This angered the human husband who then hanged himself in protest. The little boy then lived with his kin.

Here we see spirit beings taking physical form and blood infusions bringing the dead to life. A worldview of this sort is not necessarily static or bounded, but in fact is quite flexible and able to encompass or facilitate changes and ambiguities. Being essentially creative, it can comprehend analogies and differences between one situation and another or can extend itself into new circumstances, including those of contestation and conflict. Hageners in fact say that their idea of ***noman*** is a "way of speaking by comparisons" (***to tendep nitimon***). It is extensible to other "ways of speaking," and so we find in discussions of it a certain intertwining with Christian notions that were introduced into the northern part of the Hagen area from the 1950s onward and mixed with "traditional" experiential notions of self (Strathern and Stewart 1998b). Metaphorical and expressive ways of grasping the world fit well enough in general, of course, with biblical forms of expression, enabling the conflation of biblical and indigenous narratives to take place quite easily, a phenomenon found throughout New Guinea.

These flexible possibilities of extension of the self are found in many different modalities, apart from, but often interconnected with, historical changes. Three such modalities not mentioned so far are odors, clothes and decorations, and wealth items. Odors are a particularly intense part of New Guineans' imaginations of themselves: in contexts of display, for example, they use crushed herbs along with bodily decorations to project an aura of themselves and of spirit powers awakened by the occasion. Decorations, as a part of clothing, both impart their own qualities to the bodies of performers and take into themselves the residues of their wearer, becoming impregnated with the sweat or fat/grease that emerges from their skins (Strathern and Stewart 1999c). Many of the dance decorations people wear, such as plumes and shells, are themselves valuables used in exchanges, and therefore contain certain aspects of the personhood and personality of those who have worn them and given them away (Strathern and Stewart 1999b, 1999d, 2000b). Giving away a valuable, or lending it to be worn, is thus a direct transfer of a part of the donor's personal power as well as an expression of generosity, kinship, obligation, and the like. We can discern, therefore, a classic dimension of self-transfer in this expanded sensory realm of smell, bodily residues, and wealth items that reaffirms networks of personal ties and associations between people.

A further dimension of this synesthetic realm lies in people's perception of their relationship to, indeed co-identity with, aspects of their environment. Self is constantly compared with and assimilated into the outside world, as we might expect in societies where people have such a strong dependence on the environment for their livelihood and where this livelihood depends in turn on close observation and accumulation of knowledge. Thus persons and groups may be compared to plants; the humors and substances of the human body may be likened to those of plants, for example, semen and breast milk may be compared to pandanus tree sap (Herdt 1981:111 on the Sambia people); a particular humor, such as "grease," may be seen to run through humans, animals, plants, and the earth itself, as in the Melpa concept of the grease cycle (Strathern 1982; Strathern and Stewart 1999a); or people and their kinship groups may be directly equated with the ground that nourishes them and on which they, like other living things, grow, mature, and decay, an idea that is central to the worldview of the Duna people of the Southern Highlands Province of Papua New Guinea (PNG) (Stewart and Strathern 1999a, 1999b, 1999f). These forms of correspondences, partial or holistic, are very common in New Guinea, as elsewhere in the world, and they provide another reason for discerning a humoral element in their philosophies because in the ancient Greek systems of thought, for example, the elements of the universe were thought to be the same elements as those that underlie the constitution of the human body.

All of these dimensions of extension of the person are what is meant, in this context, by the term "embodiment." Bodies are both particular and general, separate from and linked to or consubstantial with others, distinct from and yet a part of the environment, different from yet indissolubly copresent with the mind of their bearers. Bodies embody both individuality and relationality, humanity as separate from other living creatures and as consubstantial with or linked to these others. Embodiment in this sense therefore implicitly covers the realm of sociality as a whole. And one of the prime bodily expressions in terms of which this expanded sense of embodiment is effected is that of food and eating. The consubstantiality of persons with their world is expressed through the growing, gathering, cooking, sharing, and consuming of food, whose substance contributes to the bodily humors (compare Knauft 1999:47; Strathern 1977a on food names). Sexual activity may be spoken of as a planting and consuming, or a fetus may be said to be "fed" by semen or nourished by blood or internal milk of the mother, so that the realm of sexuality is brought into alignment with that of feeding and the transfer of nurturant substance as a way of creating identity.

Two particularly salient features of New Guinea social relationships fall into place here: sorcery and witchcraft (Knauft 1985). Both, in one way or another, may be linked to embodiment and/or feeding. Sorcery stuff, as "poison," of course directly corresponds to an idea of "bad food," food that is rotten, has a bad smell, is associated with danger, sickness, and death. Leavings sorcery, which involves taking a part of the person and subjecting it to lethal magic, is sometimes described as an act of theft followed by a malign kind of "cooking." The Papuan novelist Vincent Eri describes a procedure from Moveave that corresponds closely to a kind of sorcery called "eaten/eating" (*nakene(a)*) in

Pangia in the Southern Highlands Province of PNG (Stewart and Strathern 1999c). Eri writes:

> [Sorcerers] collect the dirt of the person who is to die. Sometimes they cut off a piece from the person's dress. They make sure that their own dirt doesn't get on the ginger or else they are liable to die. Then they pass these things on to the experts. . . . When the mixture has been kept in a bamboo tube over a fireplace for some time, the apparition of the victim appears from time to time. The bamboo rolls about the floor when the victim is critically ill. (Eri 1976:10)

Here the heating of the mixture is like the cooking of food in a bamboo tube, a common method of cooking in Moveave, as also in Pangia and elsewhere. "Ginger" here is a general term for magical substance, seen as "hot" (powerful, dangerous).

Witchcraft is almost always conceptualized directly as an act of eating. Among the Duna the witch is said to eat the *tini* or soul of the victim (Strathern and Stewart 1999a). But the *tini* is not something immaterial. It is a part of the embodied person in the broadest sense. In fact, the witch is sometimes said to steal a victim's blood and put it into a container in a tree, then to watch over it until it "grows" into a likeness of the person, at which time it is ready to be cooked and eaten in a feast shared with other witches. Duna witches are largely thought to be mature women who have given birth to at least one child, although witchcraft itself originated with a male cannibal spirit (Strathern and Stewart 1999a). Ideas of nefarious consumption are thus linked to ideas of sexuality and to gender relations in general (see also Kelly 1976 on Etoro ideas). The notion of consumption thus joins together a number of domains in which fears of aggression are expressed. Duna witches are said to be greedy for meat or wildfowl eggs of the forest (an especially prized food source), and this greed must be appeased—people must share food. By the same token, some women become stigmatized because others fear their putative jealousy, and witchcraft fears and accusations enter into community conflicts in general, including conflicts over garden access and, thus, food resources, bringing the associations full circle from fantasy to fact.

Embodied ideas of society and relationship thus have their negative sides. Food may be poison, consumption may indicate sharing or aggression. The same symbol faces both ways. Sickness may be inflicted by sorcery and witchcraft. It may also be counteracted by healing techniques that involve the use of purges, cleansing devices, or the invocation of environmental powers metaphorically linked to the human body (Strathern and Stewart 1999a). Medicine, therefore, belongs to the same world as sorcery and witchcraft. In Chapters 2 and 3 in this volume, two contributing authors, Dianne van Oosterhout and Ien Courtens, give us further ethnographic insight into these processes, and into the concepts of human agency that stand in counterpoint to concepts of substances.

These contributions are from Irian Jaya, a province of Indonesia constituting the western half of the large island of New Guinea (see Map 1). Both peoples studied, the Inanwatan and the Ayfat, live in the Bird's Head area of Irian Jaya. We have previously conducted comparative analysis with materials from this area of New Guinea in order to look more closely at parallels with ethnographic aspects of Highlands Papua New Guinea (Strathern and Stewart 2000d).

Chapter 4 is a reflection on the materials provided from the contributions by van Oosterhout and Courtens, and a comparative exploration of similar themes from the Hagen (Melpa speakers), Duna, and Pangia (Wiru speakers) areas of the Highlands of Papua New Guinea (see Map 2).

The specific Hagen people with whom we work are the Kawelka who live at Kuk in the Wahgi Valley in the Western Highlands Province. Their main language is Melpa and many people speak Tok Pisin (pidgin English, one of the official languages of Papua New Guinea). The land where they live is fertile and suitable for growing many subsistence food crops as well as coffee and tea for sale. Pigs are extremely important and are used in bride-price and compensation payments, as well as eaten on special occasions (Strathern and Stewart 2000a).

The Duna people of the Southern Highlands are swidden-and-fallow horticulturalists who live in mountainous, forested areas that are scored by streams and lakes. The residents of the area build their dwellings on hillsides or within valley pockets at altitudes ranging from 4,000 to 6,500 feet above sea level. The region is heavily scored by limestone outcrops and sinkholes (Stewart and Strathern 1999a, 1999b).

The Pangia people of the Southern Highlands speak the Wiru language. Their area has mountain ranges on three sides. The people are horticulturalists and pig keepers, and their staple crop is sweet potato. The area has little primary forest, is mostly grassland and regrowth, and is dotted with limestone outcroppings and sinkholes (Strathern and Stewart 1999b).

All three of these PNG areas have been heavily influenced by Christian missionaries, as have the two areas from Irian Jaya discussed in Chapters 2 and 3. This point is made particularly evident in Chapter 4, in the interview materials with Anita, a Hagen female ritual expert. Also, Chapter 7 takes notice of the influence of Christian ideological thinking on indigenous ideas of the mind (***noman***) among the Hagen people, although specifying exactly how these influences have been exercised over time is a difficult task. Overall, we suggest that Christian thinking has defined and sharpened ideas of opposition between "body" and "mind/spirit" in Hagen, privileging the latter vis-à-vis the former, to some extent conflating mind with spirit, and at the same time co-opting certain notions about the interdependence of mind and body that are central to indigenous thought.

The firsthand interview materials detailed at length in Chapter 7, coming from two mature collaborators in research, strikingly underline this interdependence. Indeed, they establish ***noman*** (mind) and body/skin (***köng***) on the same existential plane by expounding how the ***noman*** is linked to head sub-

## Map 2
## Part of the Western and Southern Highlands of Papua New Guinea

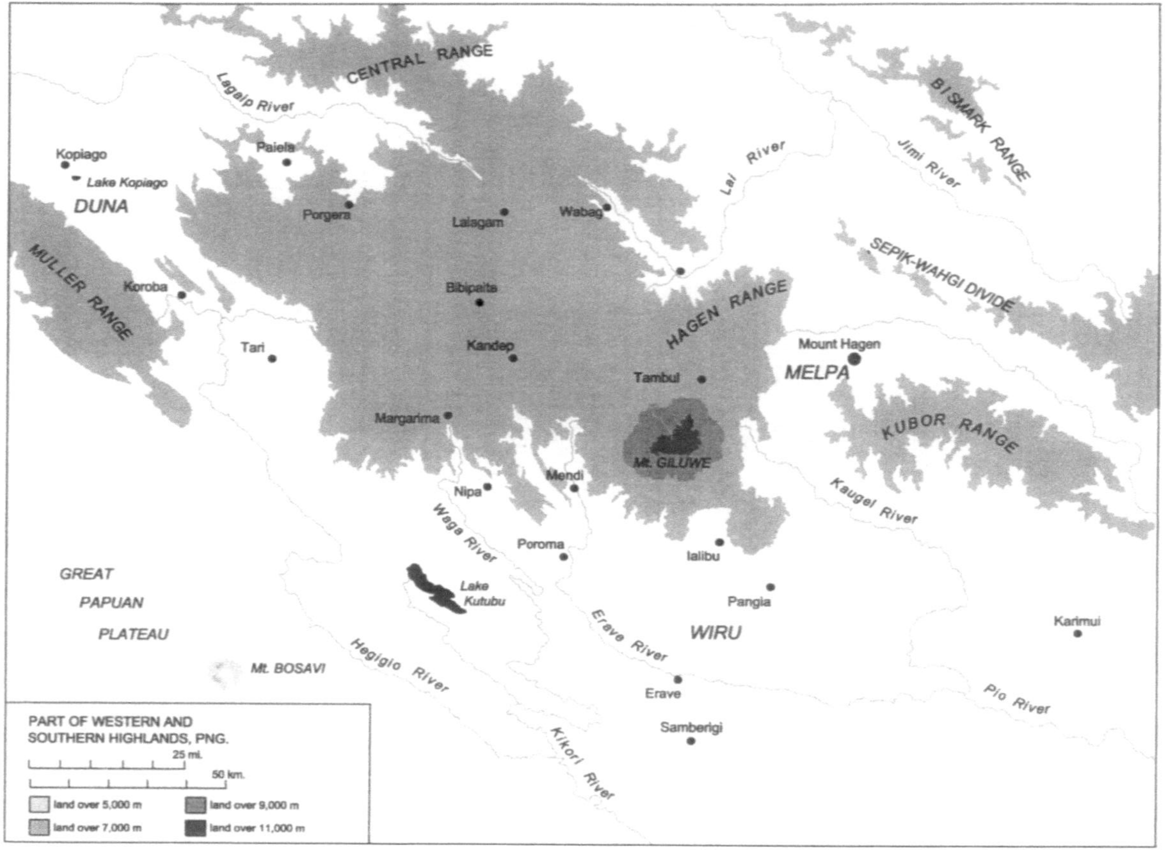

stance, spinal fluid, and reproductive fluids, such as semen and breast milk. The exposition by Wömndi, a senior Hagen man, delineates this nexus explicitly. The model Wömndi develops is largely designed to show how the elements of mind and body communicate with one another on the same plane. The mind is not so much a disembodied entity as a part of the body as a whole, even though it cannot be seen as a separate organ when the chest, where it is said to reside, is cut open. It is for this reason that we title the chapter "Mind Substance." In the interview with Ongka, another senior Hagen man, in this same chapter, Ongka slips easily from discussing the *noman* of people to discussing their *kopong* or grease: when different sorts of grease are mixed together in the reproductive act, different kinds of *noman* may emerge. Ongka's discussion therefore reinforces Wömndi's model, and, extends it into relations of gender, intermarriage, and, by implication, politics. The "grease cycle," earlier identified as important in the cosmic scheme of things (Strathern 1982; see also Strathern and Stewart 1999a), now appears to be significant also in terms of ideas of knowledge and personhood.

We may be reminded here of Raymond Kelly's discussion of the role of semen in the male initiation practices of the Etoro people of the Strickland-Bosavi region (Kelly 1976:45–53). Kelly notes that the semen orally ingested by the young initiates in cult practices was not only to make them grow physically, but also to give them personal capabilities derived from the donor of the semen. Here we see the same conjunction between "grease" and "mind" that we have found in the Hagen case, and the Hagen expression that an important leader "makes grease" (*kopong etem*) gains a further resonance from the realization that the expression joins together wealth, health, generosity, fertility, and thought. The Hagen model strongly expresses the idea that grease comes from both parents: maternal ties, however, are especially referred to as ties of blood vis-à-vis paternal ties of semen. The Etoro model also expresses one of Ongka's concerns. Ongka says that problems may come from the mixing of "incompatible" grease types. If people marry inside their own group of kin, the grease of both parents will be the same, and the *noman* of their children will stand a better chance of being harmoniously oriented. The Etoro system might be construed as a type of solution to this sort of incompatibility problem. Certainly the Etoro practices of marriage reveal a preference for restricted connubial circuits (Kelly 1977; Strathern and Stewart 2000c, 2000d).

Extending our comparative ambit a little farther, for the moment, to the Malay Peninsula, we note that the ideas of the Trengganu people reported by Carol Laderman (and commented on by Stone 1998:6) are relevant here in demonstrating the ideological connectedness of sexual fluids with mind substances. Laderman, quoting an informant's song text, reports that "for forty days and forty nights the baby rests within its father's womb [i.e. the head]" (Laderman 1991:92). Laderman refers to this as the "father's pregnancy," during which the male craves several foods. The male pregnancy is prior to the female's; she "takes over" after the father's semen thrusts the baby into her womb (Laderman 1991:ix). She tells us that "the text of the Main Peteri [a shamanic tradition of healing] clarifies Malay beliefs about the nature of men and women" (p. 92) which "date back to the time of Adam and Eve" (p. 5). She interprets the statements in this tradition to mean that "Men, however, have a greater amount of rationality than do women, in whom animal nature predominates. It makes sense, therefore, for a baby to begin life within its father's brain, the paternal womb, where it acquires rationality from a developed source" (Laderman 1991:92).

Trengganu culture appears to combine a strongly humoral set of ideas about the body with an equally strong blend of Islamic notions, including gender relations, as attested by Laderman's informants' discussion of humans, God, and angels. The informants declared that humans "are unique among God's creation in possessing the rationality (*akal*) that makes us truly human and, in this respect, even closer to God than the angels" (Laderman 1991:92). The result is something like a New Guinea theory of grease combined with "traditional" and introduced ideas of gendered hierarchy, or perhaps "identity confusion" between the roles of the sexes in conception (see Stewart and Strathern 1999d). Overall, the Trengganu model of conception as presented by Laderman would not seem entirely outlandish to New Guinea Highlanders, except that it introduces the idea of a male cerebral pregnancy rather than an overall theory of grease in the body. The Trengganu combination of Islamic theology with humoral notions of the body can also be seen in the idea that "menstruation originated when Eve ate the forbidden fruit which, because of its toxicity, turned into menstrual blood" (Laderman 1983:74). A woman is not allowed to pray while menstruating (p. 73), and Laderman says that this is because of "ritual impurity" (p. 73). She does not say that menstrual blood is considered "hot," but she indicates that conception, or the transfer of the child into the mother's womb, can occur only when both parents are in a "cool" state.

Sexual fluid, such as semen, vaginal fluids, and breast milk, has to be interpreted within an overarching set of ideas about humors and substances rather than narrowly confined to the context of sexuality itself. Rubbing semen on the body to make it grow is comparable to rubbing pork grease or healing clay on it, or sprinkling it with fresh spring water, or imbibing water, as is done in cults in Hagen and Duna (Strathern and Stewart n.d.). The same may be said of the ingestion of semen in places where the practice has been reported to occur. Semen itself can be regarded as a kind of food, both in helping a fetus to grow or come into being in the womb and after a child's birth. Transferred semen, as well as other bodily fluids, can be regarded as a general source of personal knowledge and power.

Knauft cites data on the Marind-Anim people of the south coast of New Guinea that indicate this point: relatives of a deceased person might drink the corpse's fluids in order to obtain dreams capable of disclosing "the identity of the sorcerers responsible for the death" (Knauft 1999:62, quoting Van Baal

1966:772). Moreover, novice shamans were required to ingest a dead shaman's fluids, as well as to have these rubbed into their noses and eyes, as means of obtaining the shaman's visions (Knauft 1999:62). Aspects of personality and knowledge are thus not separated off from the body but are expressed through its fluids, and the cadaveric flows are in this sense comparable to the flows of reproductive fluids, a part of the same overall cycle of renewal. The corpse's fluids contain some of the life force or "soul" of the deceased, and as this "soul" has gone into the world of the dead, it has acquired different forms of knowledge, we may suggest, that can return to the living in dreams. The nose and the eyes may also be sensory sites of experience important for shamanic knowledge generally, hence the application of fluids to them.

A similar set of ideas is expressed in the Maring people's ideas surrounding the female spirit called Kun Kaze Ambra (Smoke Woman), in which male leaders were thought to become shamans after having been "struck" by the Smoke Woman (Rappaport 1968:178). It was a relationship whereby the Female Spirit transferred knowledge between Maring men who were preparing to go to war and the ancestors known as the "red spirits," who could provide guidance. Smoke Woman mediated the ancestors' approval of the men's planned actions and an assurance of their protection for the fighters (Rappaport 1968: 119–120). Smoke Woman was specifically called upon to assist the men when the Maring were preparing for war. The way that Smoke Woman interacted with shamans was a form of possession. This occurred after the shaman had deeply and rapidly inhaled the smoke of tobacco cigars, at which time his *nomane* (spirit) was said to exit his physical body through his nose and seek out the Smoke Woman. She then returned the shaman's *nomane* to his body and slipped into his head through his nasal passages (Rappaport 1968:119; see also Strathern and Stewart 2000e). Practices of this kind, as related by Knauft and Rappaport, are tied closely both to ideas of the sensory body itself and to the wider cosmos of which it is an integral part through the channels of its own experience, its coagulations and dispersals of substances.

Reflections of this kind are relevant also to our own further discussions of "conception ideas" in relation to humors, substances, and cult ritual. Chapter 5 examines some aspects of notions of pregnancy and conception (touched on at some length also by the two Hagen men, Wömndi and Ongka, in their accounts in Chapter 7). In Chapter 5 we have a particular interest in following up questions to do with pregnancy and nurturance. Given the importance of ideas about food and substances of the body generally, it would be surprising if people did not think that pregnancy required some feeding of the child in order to make it grow. What we find in Hagen is two viewpoints. On the one hand, there is the idea that the child can perhaps grow in the womb by autophagy—as one woman put it, by "eating its own fingertips." But clearly the fingers themselves must grow by some mechanism. On the other hand, there is a notion that the child is indeed *nourished* from the mother's body, either by her blood or by milk from her breasts transmitted within the body

(Strathern and Stewart 1999a). Here nourishment can be seen as different from feeding/eating if we consider that the child in the womb is nourished directly from the mother's body.

It is significant to establish this point because the blood or grease that the mother imparts to the child is itself derived from the food she eats, and therefore from the ground on which the food is grown. Through her own body the mother imparts a physical identity to her child that is compounded of her preexisting paternal and maternal blood and of the food she has grown, prepared, and eaten on her husband's ground. The body of her child is made in this way, and so it acquires its kinship identity as a part of the whole cosmic process of fertility and reproduction of which human bodies are seen to be a part. (For a parallel in general, see Abramson 1995:199 on Fiji.) In turn, the processes of fertility in the body are mirrored by ritual acts that take place in the context of spirit cults involving both Female Spirits, who act as ritual brides, mothers, or sisters, and Male Spirits, who can make the wives of cult performers pregnant, as described in Chapter 6. Both of these spirit cult types are aimed at bringing fertility and well-being to the community at large (Strathern and Stewart 1998a). The stones that are sacred objects in these cults may be seen as objectifications of these powers of fertility. They are treated both as objects and as persons, often spoken of as the "bones" of the spirit, and their "skin" or surface is rubbed with powerful elements as decorations and as a further means of stimulating fertility and prosperity (Stewart and Strathern 1999e). Finally, cult stones are in this regard similar to the wealth items, such as shells, that are the channels for the communication and transfer of fertility between persons.

Chapter 6 considers detailed materials from a particular cult, the Wöp cult in Hagen, that has been only briefly described in earlier writings (e.g., Strathern 1970; Strathern and Stewart n.d.; see Strauss and Tischner 1962:425–435 for an ethnographic treatment in German). Apart from its cult stones, the Wöp cult was centered on water, in particular spontaneously flowing springs. Its practices perfectly symbolized the cosmic context of fertility, linking together the ritual care of the spring source, the drinking of water from it by both sexes, and the ability of the celebrant group to reproduce itself. Water in the Wöp cult was both a cosmic element and a kind of substance in the human body, and its fertility was connected with its quality of being cool and pure, like the water trapped in high-altitude mountain moss (the Melpa term for this moss is *mul-koma*, that which stays and is cool).

Cults and the desire for fertility clearly reflected the internal aims and conative wishes of people. They were tied to everyday concerns. For the Hageners they objectified these mental concerns into material practices. Chapter 7 provides an important link in the conceptualization of this relationship between what we call the mental and the material in our own cultural vocabulary by showing that the Hagen concept of the *noman* (mind) places it on a par with, and in direct interaction with, other elements of the person, such as head substance, spinal fluid, and grease (including semen and breast milk). Understanding this point is vital to the enterprise of understanding embodiment (the holistic mind–body nexus) in general among the Hageners, for example, in the realm of sickness, health, and curing practices (Strathern and Stewart 1999a).

The discussions in the various chapters are not meant to be complete ethnographies of the body and embodiment. This is partly because such discussions have appeared elsewhere, and partly because our main purpose here has been to stress the cosmic contexts in which ideas about human embodiment are given their meaning, and to show how the human mind and body are seen as transitional elements in the larger cyclicity of events. Examples of topics that are touched upon but not dealt with in depth here are medical practices (for which see Strathern and Stewart 1999a); the ethnolocations of the emotions (see Strathern 1993, 1996; Stewart and Strathern 1998; Strathern and Stewart 1998b); and the use of the terms "purity" and "pollution" in bodily contexts (see Stewart and Strathern 1999d). Also, we have not systematically discussed every aspect of the body that could be considered under the rubric of substances—for example, hair, bone, and feces—although all of these have their part in the broad conceptualizations of the body and we do mention them in the course of other discussions. Hair, for example, is a quintessential marker of growth and is accordingly important in many contexts of puberty and maturation rituals (Strathern 1989; Strathern and Stewart 1999d, n.d.), and also in magical practices. In Hagen, there was a particular emphasis in the past on the length and fullness of men's beards and on women's long ringlets. In Pangia, it was said that a woman's pubic hairs, mixed in a potion or in food, were a potent form of magic for binding the mind/inclinations (*wene*) of a sexual partner. In Duna, an infant's hair was cut at the time of naming the child by an elderly woman, known as an *Ima Ala Rao*, who possessed growth magic. This occurred around the time that the child developed its first teeth.

Bone is very widely considered to be a lasting repository of the power and identity of the person; in contrast with flesh, which rots back into the earth and thus contributes to cyclicity, bone endures and therefore may be placed in secondary burial sites as a long-term focus for commemorative sacrifice. The empty skull, devoid of its substance, was in the past still an important marker of the person in Hagen, and skull houses (*peng manga*) were built to accommodate them as a focus for ritual action. The secondary treatment of bones in this way continues among the Duna people today (Stewart and Strathern 2000). In the Duna area human bones are often kept and cared for in limestone cave shelters. In the not too distant past ancestral bones might also be kept in dwelling houses, wrapped in packets and hung from the house's roof. The belief here was that these bones could bring wealth in the form of pigs or other goods to the household members. In Pangia the bones of giant people of the high forests, associated with the sky (*akolali*) were thought to give hunting power to dogs if scrapings from them were placed in the dogs' food. Humans could dream of successful hunting and other enterprises if they slept in the high rock shelter where these bones were found. Likewise, in Duna, pulverized rodent bones were integral in marsupial hunting magic. The Duna also believed that giant cannibalistic ancestral beings (*auwape*) lived throughout the region in the past and that when they died, their ossified remains were transformed into the limestone boulders and outcroppings that mark the landscape today. Thus, the substance of these beings can be seen on a daily basis and serves as a reminder of the continuity of the past with the land and the present time.

Feces have their place in the cycle of things. For example, in the Pangia Female Spirit cult, cooked cassowary feces were rubbed onto cult stones. The cassowary is a prodigious eater of forest fruit and deposits the seeds of these through its forest ranges, helping to regenerate the wild flora. Among the Maring the spirits of the low ground (*rawa mai*) were an important counterpart to the red spirits of the mountaintops, representing fertility and regeneration (Rappaport 1968:38), and a subcategory known as *rawa tukump* were linked to rot and decay and the possibilities of contamination and sickness.

In Pangia spirits of the dead were said to frequent toilet areas and to eat the feces of humans left there, reabsorbing into the spirit realm the cast-off bodily aspects of the living. Because these same spirits controlled aspects of fertility and reproduction, it is clear that to some degree they reintegrated human feces into the overall cycle of life, death, and regeneration in this way. Yet both the dead and feces could be dangerous to humans. The dead (*ipono*) among the Pangia might "strike and eat" their human descendants (*wia nako*; reminding us here of the broader context of cannibalism) by making them sick. Forced contact with fecal materials from latrines by Pangians who were convicted of crimes and working as convicts on the colonial government station of Pangia made it necessary for those who returned from jail to purify themselves from this inappropriate contact on their return home. Again, a Pangia man killing a pig at a festival would sometimes call out *ne te moa* (you get feces!) as he clubbed the pig on its snout, a remark that was addressed to enemies or to partners thought not to reciprocate their debts, and was sometimes accompanied by actual feces expelled from the dying pig (Strathern and Stewart 1999b). Feces could therefore have inverted or negative aspects among the Pangia people: in the same vein a "feces dream" (*te pulere*) was one that depicted or predicted an event that was not to happen, including an exchange partner reneging on a promised gift (for further instances and discussion, see Clark 1995:200).

These brief examples indicate the rich and complexly ramifying associations of ideas about the body in New Guinea, sketching points on a terrain that could be mapped in greater detail. We suggest them as markers for future comparative work.

One other arena for further elaboration and comparative research is the substance transfer that takes place in dreams. We will present an example from the 1980s to illustrate the point.

### Pangia Woman Dreams of Dead Husband

A Pangia woman was pregnant and began to have dreams that involved her dead husband coming to her. He had had intercourse with her in these dreams, and she interpreted this to mean that he wanted her, and that she might die during childbirth and become a spirit. Her kinfolk were told of her dreams, and they arranged for a ritual expert to treat her with *yomberono* (magic/medicine) so that the dead husband's ghost would stop plaguing her. The condition that the woman had was a common one, and it was explained that "The spouse gave food and it went inside the skin [*tepene*], and it can get inside the *tepene* of the person again. It is *manda* [semi-formed physical essence], a light like fireflies [*taranu*] at night. A spouse may wake and see the other stretched out, hands and legs; they will die of this, or their child will die of this if the child is seen. *Manda* gets into the *tepene* or it may come to the doorway. It is the *ipono* [spirit] of dead people which comes in this way."

The ritual expert treats such a patient by laying out parsley greens on top of edible *koipo* leaves, and over this he sprinkles native salt mixed with blood from a sacrificed chicken. The woman's living husband takes some salt and ginger root, chews it, and spits it onto the greens. The mixture is then steamed and shared by the pregnant woman and others who are present, along with the *yomberono* that the ritual expert gives to the pregnant woman.

The sort of treatment described here to protect the human woman from the dead husband's taking her life force is similar to the use of *kwei* (magical leaves or smoke) among the Duna people to protect them against witches who try to kill people by taking their life force (*tini*) from them. The example here of the Pangia woman is paralled by comparable materials from both Hagen and the Duna area in which rituals were performed to appease or drive off the ghost of a man whose widow was subsequently married to another man. These rituals were likely to be performed if a dream indicated that the dead spouse was harassing the widow and might make her or her present husband sick, or kill them. In Hagen one of the pigs given by a man for a woman who was a widow and whom he was going to marry was called the *amb wöyö pol kng* (pig of the widow's bridge), and was offered to the dead husband to "eat" as a sacrifice so he would not be *wölik* (jealous). In Duna a pig was sacrificed to the ghost of a former spouse. The meat and blood from the pig were used to attract the *tini* of the dead husband into a hole on the far side of a stream, the widow being seated on the stream's near side. After the attacking *tini* had come to "eat" the pork and drink the blood, the ritual expert covered the hole with a black stone, imprisoning the dead man's *tini*. Also, in Duna when persons sleep, it is thought that their *tini* goes outside of the house, where a witch or malevolent spirit may be waiting to abduct the human's spirit, gaining power to cause the illness or death of the person unless special rituals are performed that involve the sacrifice of pigs and an offering of pork to the offending witch.

These examples indicate that although the dream world involves the actions of spirit entities and the exit of the spirit from the sleeper's body, dreams nevertheless can have physical results. This is because of the unity of the cosmos, consisting of spirit and other beings along with living humans. The same point explains the crossover between what is labeled as the metaphorical and what is labeled as the real, since reality belongs to every part of the cosmos. Humors and substances belong to the cosmos and play their vital part in its processes of maintenance and change, its stability and its flux.

## REFERENCES


Abramson, Allen. 1995. Beyond the Samoan controversy in anthropology: A history of sexuality in the eastern interior of Fiji. In Patricia Caplan, ed., *The Cultural Construction of Sexuality*, pp. 193–216. London and New York: Routledge.

Clark, Jeffrey. 1995. Shit beautiful: Tambu and Kina revisited. *Oceania* 65:195–211.

Clark, Jeffrey. 1997. State of desire: Transformations in Huli sexuality. In Lenore Manderson and Margaret Jolly, eds., *Sites of Desire, Economies of Pleasure: Sexualities in Asia and the Pacific*, pp. 191–211. Chicago: University of Chicago Press.

Csordas, Thomas (ed.). 1994. *Embodiment and Experience: The Existential Ground of Culture and Self.* Cambridge: Cambridge University Press.

Damasio, Antonio. 1999. *The Feeling of What Happens: Body and Emotion in the Making of Consciousness.* New York: Harcourt Brace.

Eri, Vincent. 1976. *The Crocodile.* Harmondsworth, UK: Penguin Books.

Foster, George M. 1994. *Hippocrates' Latin American Legacy: Humoral Medicine in the New World.* Langhorne, PA: Gordon and Breach.

Herdt, Gilbert H. 1981. *Guardians of the Flutes: Idioms of Masculinity.* New York: McGraw-Hill.

Kelly, Raymond C. 1976. Witchcraft and sexual relations: An exploration in the social and semantic implications of the structure of belief. In Paula Brown and Georgeda Buchbinder, eds., *Man and Woman in the New Guinea Highlands.* Washington, D.C.: American Anthropological Association.

Kelly, Raymond C. 1977. *Etoro Social Structure: A Study in Contradiction.* Ann Arbor: University of Michigan Press.

Knauft, Bruce M. 1985. *Good Company and Violence. Sorcery and Social Action in a Lowland New Guinea Society.* Berkeley: University of California Press.

Knauft, Bruce M. 1999. *From Primitive to Postcolonial in Melanesia and Anthropology.* Ann Arbor: University of Michigan Press.

Laderman, Carol. 1983. *Wives and Midwives: Childbirth and Nutrition in Rural Malaysia.* Berkeley: University of California Press.

Laderman, Carol. 1991. *Taming the Wind of Desire: Psychology, Medicine, and Aesthetics in Malay Shamanistic Performance.* Berkeley: University of California Press.

Lloyd, Geoffrey (ed.). 1973. *Hippocratic Writings.* Harmondsworth, UK: Penguin Books.

Meigs, Anna. 1984. *Food, Sex, and Pollution: A New Guinea Religion.* New Brunswick, NJ: Rutgers University Press.

Rappaport, Roy A. 1968. *Pigs for the Ancestors: Ritual in the Ecology of a New Guinea People.* New Haven, CT: Yale University Press.

Stewart, Pamela J., and Andrew Strathern. 1997. Sorcery and sickness: Spatial and temporal movements in Papua New Guinea and Australia. Discussion Papers Series, no. 1, pp. 1–27. Townsville, Australia: James Cook University, Centre for Pacific Studies.

Stewart, Pamela J., and Andrew Strathern. 1998. Life at the end: Voices and visions from Mt. Hagen, Papua New Guinea. *Zeitschrift für Missionswissenschaft und Religionswissenschaft* 82(4):227–244.

Stewart, Pamela J., and Andrew Strathern. 1999a. Duna landscape: Trackways, zones, cycles and transformation. *Okari Research Group Prepublication Working Paper* no. 13, pp. 1–17. Paper presented at the Dumbarton Oaks roundtable "The Cultural Production of Nature in the Tropics," Washington, DC (April 10).

Stewart, Pamela J. and Andrew Strathern. 1999b. Duna ritual trackways and movement across landscapes. *Okari Research Group Prepublication Working Paper* no. 15, pp. 1–11. Paper presented at the 4th European Society of Oceanists Conference, Leiden, Netherlands (June).

Stewart, Pamela J., and Andrew Strathern. 1999c. "Feasting on my enemy": Images of violence and change in the New Guinea Highlands. *Ethnohistory* 46(4):645–669.

Stewart, Pamela J., and Andrew Strathern. 1999d. Female spirit cults as a window on gender relations in the highlands of Papua New Guinea. *Journal of the Royal Anthropological Institute* 5(3):345–360.

Stewart, Pamela J., and Andrew Strathern. 1999e. Politics and poetics mirrored in indigenous stone objects from Papua New Guinea. *Journal of the Polynesian Society* 108(1): 69–90.

Stewart, Pamela J., and Andrew Strathern. 1999f. Time at the end: The highlands of Papua New Guinea. In Christin Kocher-Schmid, ed., *Expecting the Day of Wrath: Versions of the Millennium in Papua New Guinea,* Port Moresby, Papua New Guinea: National Research Institute.

Stewart, Pamela J., and Andrew Strathern. 2000. Naming places: Duna evocations of landscape in Papua New Guinea. *People and Culture in Oceania.* Vol. 16:87–107.

Stone, Linda. 1998. *Kinship and Gender: An Introduction.* Boulder, CO: Westview Press.

Strathern, Andrew. 1970. The female and male spirit cults in Mount Hagen. *Man* n.s. 5:571–585.

Strathern, Andrew. 1977a. Melpa food-names as an expression of ideas on identity and subsistence. *Journal of the Polynesian Society 86:503–511.*

Strathern, Andrew (trans.). 1977b. *Myths and legends from Mount Hagen.* Port Moresby: Institute of Papua New Guinea Studies.

Strathern, Andrew. 1982. Witchcraft, greed, cannibalism, and death. In Maurice Bloch and Jonathan Parry, eds., *Death and the Regeneration of Life*, pp. 111–133. Cambridge: Cambridge University Press.

Strathern, Andrew. 1989. Flutes, birds, and hair in Hagen (PNG). *Anthropos* 84:81–87.

Strathern, Andrew. 1993. Organs and emotions: The question of metaphor. *Canberra Anthropology* 16(2):1–16.

Strathern, Andrew. 1996. *Body Thoughts.* Ann Arbor: University of Michigan Press.

Strathern, Andrew, and Pamela J. Stewart. 1998a. Embodiment and communication: Two frames for the analysis of ritual. *Social Anthropology* 6(2):237–251.

Strathern, Andrew, and Pamela J. Stewart. 1998b. Seeking personhood: Anthropological accounts and local concepts in Mount Hagen, Papua New Guinea. *Oceania* 68(3):170–188.

Strathern, Andrew, and Pamela J. Stewart. 1999a. *Curing and Healing: Medical Anthropology in Global Perspective.* Durham, NC: Carolina Academic Press.

Strathern, Andrew, and Pamela J. Stewart. 1999b. Outside and inside meanings: Non-verbal and verbal modalities of agonistic communication among the Wiru of Papua New Guinea. *Man and Culture in Oceania* 15:1–22.

Strathern, Andrew, and Pamela J. Stewart. 1999c. Self-decoration in Hagen and Hagu (Papua New Guinea): Display and disjuncture. Paper presented at the session "Embodying Modernity and Postmodernity in Melanesia," organized by Sandra Bamford. 98th Annual Meeting, American Anthropological Association, Chicago.

Strathern, Andrew, and Pamela J. Stewart. 1999d. *"The Spirit Is Coming!" A Photographic–Textual Exposition of the Female Spirit Cult Performance in Mt. Hagen.* Ritual Studies Monograph Series, no. 1. Pittsburgh: University of Pittsburgh, Department of Anthropology.

Strathern, Andrew, and Pamela J. Stewart. 2000a. *Arrow Talk: Transaction, Transition, and Contradiction in New Guinea Highlands History.* Kent, Ohio: Kent State University Press.

Strathern, Andrew, and Pamela J. Stewart. 2000b. Dangerous woods and perilous pearl shells: The fabricated politics of a longhouse in Pangia, Papua New Guinea. *Journal of Material Culture* 5(1):69–89.

Strathern, Andrew, and Pamela J. Stewart. 2000c. Kinship and commoditization: Historical transformations. *L'Homme* no. 154–155:373–390.

Strathern, Andrew, and Pamela J. Stewart. 2000d. *The Python's Back: Pathways of Comparison Between Indonesia and Melanesia.* Westport, CT: Bergin and Garvey.

Strathern, Andrew, and Pamela J. Stewart. 2000e. Rappaport's Maring: The challenge of ethnography. In M. Lambek and E. Messer eds., *Thinking and Engaging the Whole: Essays on Roy Rappaport's Anthropology.* Ann Arbor: University of Michigan Press.

Strathern, Andrew, and Pamela J. Stewart. n.d. Cults, closures, and collaborations. For a volume containing a collection of papers from the "Women in Male Rituals of New Guinea" session, convened by Pascale Bonnemère, at the 1999 ASAO (Association for Social Anthropology in Oceania) meeting, Hilo, Hawaii.

Strauss, Hermann, and Herbert Tischner. 1962. *Die Mi-Kultur der Hagenberg Stämme.* Hamburg: Cram, de Gruyter.

Van Baal, J. 1966. *Dema.* The Hague: Martinus Nijhoff.

Vicedom, Georg F., and Herbert Tischner. 1943. *Die Mbowamb.* Vol. 3, *Mythen und Erzählungen.* Hamburg: Friederichsen, de Gruyter.

Zimmerman, Francis. 1982. *The Jungle and the Aroma of Meats: An Ecological Theme in Hindu Medicine.* Berkeley: University of California Press.

# CHAPTER 2

# The Scent of Sweat: Notions of Witchcraft and Morality in Inanwatan

*Dianne van Oosterhout*

In Inanwatan, a south coastal Bird's Head society in Irian Jaya (Indonesia), humoral ideas of the body are focused predominantly on the balance of blood. Imbalance is revealed by the foul scent of the body, excreted via the skin through sweat. This scent may easily attract spirit attacks, but is foremost interpreted as a sign of ill health and immorality. An important way to restore the balance of blood is through purification—for instance, by causing excessive sweat. In this essay I will show how a foul scent of the body influences an individual's position in society and directs the actions undertaken when pollution is diagnosed. Because a bad scent may indicate witchcraft (locally called *suangi*), patients are experienced as a threat to society. I will first briefly discuss the sociocultural context in which humoral ideas of the body are interpreted, a context in which notions of decay and loss of life force are predominant. Then I will focus on the connotations of bodily fluids in Inanwatan, particularly on witchcraft as a form of substance exchange. Finally, I will show how the purification methods used for moral illnesses are based on the excretion of polluting substances and their transfer to other bodies or domains.

## PROCESSES AND EVALUATION OF CHANGE IN INANWATAN

Inanwatan is located in the coastal mangrove swamps that stretch along the southern part of the easternmost province of Indonesia (Irian Jaya). This geographical and environmental setting influences the health of the population. The moist swamps, for instance, are, the habitat of various types of mosquitoes, which transmit endemic malaria, and fungi, which cause skin diseases. The local infrastructure is still relatively basic, compared with the central part of the Indonesian state, particularly in terms of transportation and health facilities. Patients are therefore mostly dependent on indigenous healers and home remedies. This does not mean, however, that Inanwatan is particularly isolated. The population maintains trade and marriage relationships with other ethnic groups living in the interior of the peninsula or along the coastline, and a considerable part of the Inanwatan population resides for long periods of time in the nearest town, Sorong, where they come in contact with migrants from other Indonesian provinces. Furthermore, trade contacts with other parts of eastern Indonesia have taken place over an extended period of time; in particular with middlemen and *raja-raja* (rulers, local "kings") from the Bird's Head Peninsula, the southern Onin Peninsula, and the Moluccas (Haga 1884: II, 307–308). Through these trade relations, diverse products, other languages and ethnic groups, as well as Islam, were introduced into the area, (Haga 1884: I, 290). Since the end of the nineteenth century, small groups of traders from China, and later from Sulawesi (Celebes) have settled permanently in Inanwatan. Missionaries from the Moluccas and western Europe, and Dutch colonial administrators followed them during the second decade of the twentieth century introducing Christianity and Western health care, and initiating village formation. Inanwatan was initially formed from seventeen *gobo* (river arm, "clan" domains) spread around the mangrove wetlands. In the 1960s Irian Jaya became part of the Indonesian state, a fact that continues to have an impact on its social and spatial outlook. The population of Inanwatan has remained remarkably stable—from around 1500 at its foundation to less than 2000 at present—despite the high birth rate and decreased death rate. This is mainly the result of out-migration by young people, who settle in Sorong to look for better opportunities.

Recent developmental plans, such as a land connection to Sorong, the construction of a village marketplace, and the settlement of an oil company should improve the economic opportunities within Inanwatan, and hence improve local standards of living. Although most of my informants saw the advantages of such events, they did not really expect to profit from them. Many informants said that the benefits would surely go to outsiders, and that exploitation of the land would disturb the cosmological balance and eventually destroy all life.

Although Christianity is perceived as a possible way to maintain or restore this balance, the church was believed to be hiding its deepest knowledge, and thus denying the local population a route to development or salvation. The relationship between the local population and the church is ambivalent because, on the one hand, Christianity is deeply integrated within Inanwatan life, yet on the other hand, its representatives appear to condemn local expressions of Christianity and attempt to purify them. Furthermore, the local idea of an approaching end of time that is caused by immoral behavior not only parallels Christian visions and is likely to be influenced by them, but is also distanced by the (Biak) vicars. The latter stress that one is never sure when this will happen. Destructive floods followed by a new order formed a dominant theme in local myths collected in the early days of pacification, and found a new impulse in Christian doctrine, but the vicars' refusal to provide certainty was interpreted as either a purposeful denial of salvation to the local population or as a kind of test to single out true believers. This kind of ambiguity, as we will see later, plays a role in defining the borders between "good" and "evil," between God and *suangi* (witch), when the end comes near.

Intriguingly, Inanwatan concepts of the body and notions of scent can help to explain local perceptions of development and expectations of the nearing end. When I asked how to define Inanwatan identity, I often was given the answer:

> We all share the same food, and therefore the same flesh and scent[1]; we have the same origins and share the same blood.

Shared origins and shared substance define Inanwatan identity. Although each *gobo* possesses a different version of history, the histories of other *gobo* are perceived as part of the same truth, like another branch from the same tree of origins. Therefore all *gobo* share the same bodily substances, have the same blood running through their bodies. The experience of decay is also expressed in terms of bodily substances: bodies have grown smaller and skinnier; blood has become less fluid, less strong, and more polluted; and skins have become more flaccid and dirty. A decreased fluidity of blood is identified as the major cause of these bodily changes, and is, in turn, perceived to be caused by a disturbed relationship with ancestors and the land, the domain of origins. Christianization is identified as part of the cause of these disturbances, because "people were urged to forget the ways of their ancestors." The question remains how fluidity of blood enhances bodily strength or even social well-being. People move in time and space, they are dynamic and fluid. Through marriage and death their juices flow from *gobo* to *gobo*, where they enter new bodies, and from bodies to the earth, and back again in the form of food.[2] They connect different groups of people, and people to their land, in a constant process.

By contrast, the ancestors and the domain or tree of origins, conceptualized as both a woman and a tree (called *Kekea'o*), are identified as the hard, enduring core or "bones" of society. This core is perceived as a source of life force or potency, locally called *iware*, which encompasses health, strength, power, success, sacral knowledge, creativity, growth, and procreation. When people trespass taboos, or refrain from giving proper return gifts, the core may withhold *iware* from them. This is clearly present in myths about floods, the first major depleting occurrence in which the core takes revenge for the actions of human beings. Whereas people formerly were part of an encompassing "body," they became separated through their sexual greed. Disappointed, *Kekea'o* went westward, taking most secret knowledge (*iware*) with her and leaving her descendants bereft of their most important source of *iware*. This depletion of *iware* led to attempts to control the remaining *iware*, causing accumulation or depletion. Such depletion provides us with an answer to the experience of decreasing strength or well-being; obviously depleted *iware* causes decreasing health and strength. Healing therefore centers on restoring the flow of *iware* (e.g., through enhancing the fluidity of blood).

On a different level the same principle is used: social obstruction or decay is treated by stimulating the flow of people's "blood," for instance by making communal offerings. Furthermore, the notion of a depletion of *iware* has probably influenced the way in which external elements have been integrated. Because new, influential people (including missionaries) came *from the west*, their artifacts, languages, customs, and ideas were experienced as expressions of a power derived from a powerful source and, more important, as a sign that they were perhaps close descendants of Kekea'o. Some informants suggested that their ancestors thought accommodating these innovations would provide them with access to the source. Furthermore, various informants said that the vicars and drillers knew quite well what they were here for: not just to teach Christianity or drill for oil, but in fact to find the domain of origins and capture the sacral source of *iware*. Their superficial aims were explained as a mere masquerade; their "tools" (*guci* [vessels], the Bible, machines) probably hide a deeper secret. By mastering these tools, then, it would be possible to grasp their real meaning and regain access to *iware*. However, as already noted, most informants no longer believed these secrets would ever be revealed to them, and had lost hope of external agencies being willing to help them retrieve what was lost.

The concern with depleted *iware* and the experienced lack of participation in development is therefore related to morality; the acquisition and division of *iware* is regarded as essentially a moral problem. In the following sections I focus on various bodily substances and show how these substances contain or transport *iware*, encode meanings and moral statements. These can in principle be read on the skin, but individuals can use deception to hide their inner bodies. Scent proves to be the only way to reveal the true inner state of a person or even of society at large. Finally, I will show how purification and deception are used to restore the moral flow of *iware*.

## THE SCENT OF DEPLETION

Blood has to flow fluently in order to preserve the flow of *iware*. Exchange objects such as *guci* have long been the motor to keep this flow going. Such *guci* contain a soul (*sombar, ara'ugo*) to replace the new life the ancestors and progenitors provide, which makes them suitable exchange gifts. But what really matters is the resultant fluidity, not so much how this is attained. Fluidity functions as a dividing device, circulating and dividing *iware* along a chain of relationships. This is related to the concept of a closed, bounded system in which the total amount of *iware* is circulating,[3] although in practice depletion is indeed possible through escaping or destroyed *iware*. Polluted blood, for instance, slows and thickens, causing an obstruction of the flow. *Iware* becomes immobile, leading to depleted life force, and illness or death. Objects and spirits may now easily intrude into and reach its core because it is no longer encompassed by the circulation of blood.

Obstruction of the flow in this way also leaves room for the core to "escape," which is exactly what happened when *Kekea'o* left. Not surprisingly, this departure is compared to what happens when flesh is separated from its bones. The juices stop flowing, the spirit leaves, and the flesh starts to decompose, eventually laying bare the bones. Typically, the remnants of *Kekea'o,* which stayed behind when she left, are described as a dry and hollow tree through which the juices have stopped running. Its bark (skin) is wrinkled and rough, and its core (bones) is empty.[4] The remnants of houses or machines are also lifeless and empty because *iware* has stopped flowing. In most cases, the depleted *iware* enters a different body or element, and is thus secured for recirculation. However, when rotting starts before the actual death, *iware* leaves the body prematurely (out of time) and publicly (out of place), instead of after death and in isolation, and hence causes obstruction or depletion of its flow.

It is particularly in this process of premature rotting that scent plays an essential role in Inanwatan concepts of bodily health and fertility and the well-being of society. The hidden process of rotting will be revealed on the skin, and the foul scent reveals what is taking place below the surface. This scent may, for instance, attract spirit attacks, but it also indicates illness and immorality. Persons with a rough and bad skin are, for instance, suspected of stealing. We have already seen that bodily substances or processes taking place in the body can function to describe relationships between people and their origins. This is also valid for other relationships, such as those of gender, kinship, and trade. Marx compared various studies conducted in Papua New Guinea and Irian Jaya, and came to the conclusion that

> Ideas about gender and relations between women and men in New Guinea cultures are largely couched in terms of bodily substances, their manipulation, and their interpersonal transfer. (Marx 1994:10)

In a similar manner, the perceived decay of Inanwatan society is explained as an obstruction of the flow of blood (exchange relations) and as premature rotting of its "flesh" (the immoral conduct of members of society). Its symptoms are visible on the "skin," in the form of diminished prosperity and autonomy, increased marital violence, and increased use of invisible forces such as black magic (*ilmu hitam*) or witchcraft (*suangi*).[5] These are expressions of disorder or loss of control, of the "dirty laundry" of a society, and are often talked of in terms of *bau* (smell): *dorang bau ilmu* (they smell of black magic) or *dong bau bras* (they smell of rice, implying they are associated with the Indonesian government, and hence with greed).

Scent, being a bodily substance, is a communicative essence. It functions as a platform on which relationships can be expressed, on the level of the individual body and also in society. Loudon defined this function as follows:

> Some of the [shed] substances are commonly employed as indicators of the organism's relationship with the environment, whether internal or external, social or physical; they also play an important part in the expression and communication of ideas. (Loudon 1977:162)

The scent of sweat is more than just pleasant or oppressive; it conveys a message of decay and illness, or of *iware* and health. Scent is associated with trespassing taboos, and consequently with pollution or prematurely rotting flesh. Scent is thus excreted through substances that are "out of place" or "out of time." In a recent article on Highland Papua New Guinea, P. J. Stewart and A. Strathern point out the polluting effect of something out of place, in this case menstrual blood. They regard pollution as "identity confusion" (1997b:10): "Menstrual blood out of its Douglasian place reverses the proper order of fertility and can be destructive" (Stewart and Strathern 1997b:22). Scent, in Inanwatan, also says something about processes taking place within the body that are related to conduct out of place or out of time, to immoral conduct that reverses the normal order. Scent is a residue or expression of relations, a foul scent being an expression of disturbed relations or immoral conduct. The entire body is, you could say, a display of relations with other people, with the communal land, or with the ancestors. It is a microcosm of relations.[6] These relationships are, in Inanwatan, most clearly exposed on the skin.

The skin forms the mediating link between the inner body and the outside world; it also separates them, thus defining their boundaries. The skin is permeable; internal substances can be excreted and vice versa. Concerning the mobility of body parts and the function of the skin, M. Strathern noted:

> Such parts or appendages can also be objects outside the boundary of the skin, yet are nevertheless considered part of the person. The perception of Melanesian bodies as internally divided creates an apparent homology between internal and external relations or parts. Thus the person, "composed of relations," appears to extend beyond the skin boundary to include objects and persons considered at any one time to be an objectification of such relations. It is easy to see then how transactions appear as the extraction, and absorption, of parts of the person. In being multiple it is also partible, an entity that can dispose of parts in relation to others. (M. Strathern 1988:185)

Scent, as an objectification of relations, is in Inanwatan considered transferable as well. It exposes a part of the body (polluted substance), and is both produced in relation to others and exposed in relation to others. It follows that a person's scent may be absorbed into another body through the skin. The shedding of scent therefore invites and necessitates a reaction from others.

In Inanwatan, sweat is considered an important way to transport polluted substance, and this principle therefore plays an important role in purification methods, including the purification of scent. Sweat is a (fluid) visualization of scent. It contains scent in condensed form as opposed to gastric forms of substances, which explains why sweat and scent are often associated with one another. However, it should be noted that scent can be shed without visible sweat and that sweat does not necessarily excrete a foul scent. Sweat is defined as smelling bad only if it is related to ailments or illness and to the shedding of polluted substances. Perspiration caused by the sun or by engaging in physical labor, for instance, does not smell foul, even though dirt may come out with it.

Food may likewise cause perspiration, particularly sago porridge (whereas baked sago does not). The first step in new sago exchange relationships is therefore formed by gifts of baked sago. Causing sweat would not be a proper way to start a relationship, because it causes embarrassment to both parties; even though the scent of "sago-sweat" is in principle considered pleasant, it is *potentially* foul, and thus avoided. The causes of sweating are diverse: health, labor, intercourse, food, polluted blood, or rotting flesh. Whenever it is shed out of place or out of time, sweat will excrete a foul scent. Sweat as such keeps a body healthy by promoting the fluidity of blood, and therefore plays an important role in healing. Polluted substance, including scent, thus finds a way out, and the moisture keeps the skin shiny. However, excessive sweat drains fluid from the body, and could therefore threaten the fluidity of blood. Sweat can thus disturb or promote the balance of bodily humors, and can contain polluted essence in the form of a foul scent. It should therefore be shed in a controlled manner.

Sweat plays a role in healing as well as in illness classification: it both exposes and evacuates scent. We saw that the body, in Inanwatan, functions as a metaphor expressing processes taking place in society. Like a body, society can be polluted or decaying, and its excrements are likewise visible on the surface, for instance, in the form of sweat (floods). In a larger context, then, scent says something about the moral state of the community as a whole, whereas in relation to other people, it defines identity and moral value. Scent is therefore both a way to define outsiderhood and to deal with an inability to protect the core of society or share in development. To understand the meaning of scent in Inanwatan, and how scent is dealt with, we first have to understand more about the connotations of blood, flesh, and boundaries between bodies (skin), and what role they have in exchange relationships. Scent is but one possible expression of these relationships, but it is a substance which is intrinsically related to morality.

## THE SCENT OF FLESH AND BLOOD

The soft, fluid parts of the body are released after death. They enter the soil and feed the vegetation. Eventually, it is believed, these transformed soft body parts reenter the body as food, and are stored in the form of flesh and blood. Through nurturance the body is shaped and modeled. The care invested in an individual by others is revealed in body shape; social relations are thus expressed through body shape. An elderly informant described this as follows:

> Look how skinny I am. I am only bones with some skin, I have little flesh left. You know, I have given birth to many children and I have worked for them until my bones hurt. But who is taking care of me now? I don't need much, but my son, he does not give me anything, his wife does not let him.

Her skinny body is a public message to the community of her marginalized position and of the shortcomings of her close relatives. The amount of flesh on a body symbolizes the intensity of care in the form of nurture invested in the individual.[7] In Becker's words, the body "reflects the achievements of its caretakers" (1995:57). It is the locus of vested efforts. Flesh is therefore not an individual matter, but a social one. Failure to invest in the flesh of nurture relations could lead to suspicions of greediness, of an unwillingness to share and nurture, or of excessive individuality. The volume of flesh is thus a moral judgment of a person's capability to maintain proper relationships.[8] A *suangi* fails to share food, and steals the flesh and blood of others. He or she negates exchange both by withholding *nurturing* substance (food) and by stealing *nurtured* substance (flesh).

In a similar way, in Papua New Guinea "people are judged 'good' or 'bad' according to whether they share or hoard food" (Kahn 1986:37). Sharing food, then, is in Inanwatan an essential element in expressing good intentions. However, this practice also forms an easy medium to enact grievances. By supplying food of low quality, for instance, a person meets the demand of sharing, but at the same time is able to show resentments. In addition, food forms a perfect medium for poisoning, which helps explain why gifts of food are always carefully examined, and why exchange relationships do not easily cross kinship borders. Flesh is thus primarily formed by close kin who provide proper food, that is, food from their own gardens. If people say, then, that they have the same flesh, they mean that they have eaten from the same land. Their flesh is formed by the same food. Through the consumption of food from their own gardens, spilled ancestral substance (containing *iware*) reenters the body and contributes to its flesh (and *iware*):

> We, the grandchildren, eat the sago our ancestors have planted. That is why sago of other people does not taste any good, we cannot eat it. Their ancestors will get angry and make us ill. We can only eat from our own ancestors. They planted and fed the trees. We are made out of sago.

Because sago is the main staple food in Inanwatan, flesh is mainly constructed by the consumption of sago. Bloch and Parry described a similar concept for the Melanesian Dobu in relation to yams:

> The flesh in the Dobuan idiom is planted in the gardens as the corpses of the ancestors are planted in the village mound. What reproduces the lineage in a material sense, then, is—in Dobuan ideology—the flesh of its own kind. The consumption of yams . . . thus amounts to an act of symbolic endo-cannibalism. (Bloch and Parry 1982:28)

Consuming flesh of their own thus contributes to the construction of flesh of their own in the following generations. This explains why (planted) sago should not be eaten by strangers. But there is more to it. The processing and consumption of sago is often used in a metaphorical sense to refer to sexual acts and consequent conception.

Sharing sago therefore has some sexual connotations, which in turn has implications for kinship and avoidance rules. The main nurturers within a kin group are the paternal uncles; they give most food to their brothers' children. They have raised their brothers' daughters, and therefore receive the largest share of bride-price payments. Since parallel cousins are thus fed by the same sago, and also share the same flesh, they are like siblings and cannot marry; this would be incest.[9] Married women cannot eat with the father and uncles of their husbands, who are "of the same flesh," and have to avoid them until they have grown children of their own. Although they now share food from the same gardens, they cannot consume it communally, and may even eat from separate trees. A woman becomes a full member of her husband's community only when she is allowed to eat *with* them (and from the same tree) instead of *from* them. Only then her scent is considered to be the same as her in-laws'.

This seemingly small detail has some serious implications, because it partly explains why in-married women are more often prone to *suangi* accusations than others. Until a wife has returned the investments her husband's relatives have made in terms of wealth and food, she is considered to be a parasite who merely consumes, and hence potentially a *suangi*. Her husband and his relatives are in turn perceived to be the easiest victims of *suangi* attacks.

The consumption of food thus has implications for the construction of familiar flesh as opposed to unfamiliar flesh, for exchange and avoidance rules, and for familiar and unfamiliar scent. Semen is a major producer of *new* flesh (as opposed to "more of the same"). It coagulates with female blood. The fetus is thus partly constructed out of familiar substance and partly out of foreign substance. Through sharing the same food, the child gradually becomes more of the same flesh. In addition, boys used to be nurtured by oral insemination of semen (i.e., giving them more *iware*) to make them grow faster and stronger.[10] The boys were fed by their paternal uncles, who thus contributed to their growth in the form of food and semen.[11] This focus on nurture could be seen in the context of constructing "flesh of one's own" and "scent of one's own," as opposed to female nurture in the form of breast milk and female blood. The male child gradually becomes more of the same flesh.

Through nurturance, then, *iware* in the form of blood, semen, scent, and flesh is transferred between different generations and descent groups. Scent is inherited along with blood and flesh. These substances are mobile, but this mobility is regulated according to strict rules. Substances moved to the wrong category (for instance, to tabooed relationships) are considered substances "out of place." Hunchbacks and bulges or tumors are examples of such substance out of place, caused by clotting of blood in the wrong context. Transfers "out of time" are especially associated with scent; a man who has ejaculated in a taboo period will have weak flesh that smells bad. This does not necessarily make him a *suangi*, however, and the resultant scent may be detectable only by spirits. A *suangi* has *illegally* consumed the flesh, blood, or semen of living human beings, and therefore possesses plentiful and foul-smelling flesh. By contrast, consuming flesh of bodies killed in battle is not defined as *suangi* but as a kind of growth medicine, as enhancing a person's *iware*. Consuming or transferring substance in the proper context, then, is considered as constructing flesh of one's own, whereas other transfers cause bad-smelling flesh, a scent that is released through the skin.

Blood, like flesh, is related to its context. Blood transfer in the process of conception, for instance, is not considered out of place, and is therefore not threatening and does not produce a bad smell. If blood is polluted, however, it will certainly smell bad, and its scent is released through sweat. Polluted blood may also be shed through wounds or, on purpose, through incisions. Sweating sheds polluted substance without blood, which is rather different. Polluted blood from wounds or incisions is primarily defined by color and temperature. Blood transports polluted substance and is affected by other polluted or polluting substances. It ideally flows fluently and is neither too hot nor too cold. Pollution usually makes the blood hotter, whereas spirit attack occasionally makes it colder. Both extremes cause ill health. Hot blood flows very fast and therefore clots easily, causing obstruction of its flow. Cold blood is associated with shivering and old age. It is lighter than hot blood, and flows more slowly.

The central Bird's Head Mejprat likewise distinguish hot and cold blood, and relate this distinction to gender: cold blood is associated with, among other things, maleness, death, and action, whereas hot blood is associated with femininity, the power of growth, and passivity (see Elmberg 1968:208). Some similar associations between heat and passivity (slow) and cold and activity (fast) are made in Inanwatan, but both sexes may possess hot or cold blood. Healthy blood is thus warm and fluid. It is also strong. The strength of blood varies: young persons generally possess stronger and hotter blood than others. Strong blood contains much *iware*, whereas in weak blood, *iware* has been depleted. The amount of *iware* in the blood can legally be enhanced by controlled consumption:

> Before there were vitamins, we ate red ferns to strengthen the blood. During head-hunting raids they used to eat each other. Then we were taller and stronger indeed.

Usually taboos are explained as preventing the heating of blood. Possessing *ilmu* ("knowledge"), for instance, or marrying too closely heats the blood. In local illness etiology, hot blood causes various health problems, whereas weak blood negatively influences bodily growth and strength. When circulation is obstructed and blood clots out of time or place, it can result in pollution and flesh out of place:

You must think the body of a human being is like a sago tree. We are like a sago tree. Through this tree there also run fluids. If the roots are stuck, then it cannot flow fluently. It is like that with the blood of people. If there is an obstruction, it cannot flow fluently and you get ill. The dirt piles up. Then you can get wild flesh.

Such flesh is uncontrolled, as opposed to the cultivated flesh constructed by nurture. In a similar manner, uncontrolled desire causes pollution of blood and hence obstruction of the flow of blood, or clotting out of place. Such bad blood emits a foul scent.

This brings us yet again to *suangi*. Its greed for food causes consumption out of place. Female *suangi* can negate exchange by magically stealing semen from men, or by displaying too much desire. This semen clots with her blood, producing a child "out of place." Desire for blood is also a mark of a *suangi*, who, magically or literally, consumes the blood of people, thus strengthening its blood without a countergift. It possesses blood "out of place," but this does not affect its health, as it would a normal person's. This seems to me an example of what Stewart and Strathern defined as "identity confusion" (1997b:10). The immoral conduct of *suangi* does not affect health or skin, as in normal people, and they thus "confuse" others about their real identity. However, they give themselves away by their foul scent.

## SKIN, SCENT, AND MORALITY

The skin forms the boundary between the body and society, and is dynamic and fluid in relation to the outside world. The skin covers the flesh, blood, and bones, so only the shape, volume, and strength of the body are visible. The internal dynamics of the body, such as the flow of blood, food consumption, and the production of sexual fluids, are obscured. In Inanwatan it is said that you can "read" the skin and thus obtain information about that hidden state of the body:

You can see the inner state of a person from the skin. A thief betrays himself in this way. Some people put oil on their skin to make it beautiful. A skin smells of blood. If the blood is dirty, the skin will smell bad.

A bad skin is thus associated with misconduct and with polluted blood. Typically, a bad skin smells foul. This smell carries an additional message. It conveys poor health or misconduct, such as eating tabooed food or transgressing sexual taboos.

In other parts of New Guinea, the relationship between bad skin and misconduct is made in a similar manner. In Waghi, for instance, betrayal of fellow clansmen is revealed in a flaccid skin (O'Hanlon 1989:68). Bad skin, in turn, generates infertility and death, implying that traitors would not be able to produce offspring. In Inanwatan the relationship between skin and fertility is similar. Old people, for instance, have a dry and flaccid skin, and are no longer capable of reproduction. Women with a bad skin are more often prone to accusations of *suangi* than others, particularly if they are childless. Bad skin and infertility are seen as proof of *suangi* identity, even though, confusingly, a *suangi* is said to be able to hide his or her "real" skin. This contradiction is not explained, but I surmise that it is due to a tension between concept and practice, a tension that makes *suangi* comprehensible and intangible at the same time. It is part of a deliberate "identity confusion." Conversely, someone with a beautiful skin is perceived to be a good and fertile person; the skin reveals the possession of *iware*. Bad skin and foul scent always initiate interpretations of their cause, and usually the behavior of the afflicted is scrutinized.

This makes the skin a perfect platform for explicating or interpreting social relations; through the skin the social connectedness of a person may be revealed.[12] Antisocial behavior such as stealing, hoarding, breaching taboos, or self-isolation is believed to be revealed on the skin. The quality of the skin is thus socially produced; it is the result of social relations. In a similar way, O'Hanlon states that bodies and skins do not occur naturally, but are seen as "the outcome of the state of specific social relationships" (1989:138). The skin, as already indicated, is like a membrane between the body and society, where messages can be explicated or internalized. Through the skin the inner state, such as pollution or morality, is excreted and exposed on the surface, where it can be interpreted and taken into consideration in social relationships. The skin is thus a mirror of the inner body, a medium that makes a hidden dimension visible.[13] This hidden dimension is primarily the moral conduct embodied in flesh and blood. In this line of thought, then, it is very hard to cover this hidden dimension, and sooner or later a person will give himself or herself away—unless he or she is very clever at the art of deception.

In Inanwatan there are several ways to make oneself invisible or to "empty" the skin (*kulit kosong*; empty skin, skin without messages). Therefore, a *suangi* may *appear* to be an innocent child or beautiful woman (i.e., purposeful "confusing identity"). In contacts with related people, such deception is unacceptable. You should show your real skin. Disclosure of the skin is even used to prove moral rightness; in a fight, for instance, people tear off their clothes and point out that they have nothing to hide. When the first vicars settled in the area, this led to considerable confusion because they portrayed themselves as messengers from God but they dressed like people who had to hide something. An informant explained:

> My grandparents did not trust them, they were dressed from head till toe. They said they could not read them, could not tell who they were, if they could be trusted. One of them was considered to be a dangerous *suangi*. He said he could cure people, but nobody dared to trust him. I think that the other vicars wanted to hide their power so they could secretly look for Kekea'o.

In this narrative we see that the vicars' clothing was ambiguously interpreted, following the various perceptions of their real intentions. Occasionally, however, deception is believed to be used as a test. People with very bad skin may have "put it on" (i.e., purposeful "identity confusion") to test and guard the morality of society. God (or Are Iware [He who creates]), for instance, is described as a very old man with dry, ugly, and smelly skin who begs for food. He is the typical example of someone negating exchange. Only people with true knowledge of *iware* would be able to see through this disguise. Deception may even be admired, as in the case of fooling an enemy until he believes himself safe, so that one can strike even more vengefully. The trick is not showing one's real (bad) intentions.

The skin thus forms a stage for both deception and counterdeception, for both involuntary and purposeful disclosure (as in enhancing beauty). On the one hand, *iware* is revealed (as in a fight) or suggested (*suangi*), and on the other hand, *iware* is hidden (God). There are thus several possible layers, hidden below others or revealed on top of others, some permitted or even admired, and others prohibited. In a paper on deception among the Huli, Goldman describes "a stream of deceitful interaction" that is arranged on two intersecting axes, one involving morality:

> One axis describes the continuum of inventiveness: from creative political lies to the preformulated and routinized deception in children's games, religious rituals, or culturally shaped caretaker-child interaction. The second cross–cutting axis defines perceptions of the action as permitted, prescribed, or prohibited. (Goldman 1995:117)

A *suangi*'s deceit would then be defined as a prohibited, creative political lie, whereas deceiving an enemy would be permitted and even preformulated. This concept helps to explain why a *suangi* has bad skin, but may use deceit to cover it under a false skin. It also helps to explain why, initially, the vicars' appearance led to confusion; it did not clearly fall into known categories. Goldman further argues that the point of deceit is that "the medium of deceit is the message" (1995:137). In this case, then, the skin itself would be the message. In other words, the skin may both hide and reveal the truth.

As a membrane, the skin absorbs external substances, such as poisons, objects, and the polluting substance of others. In this way the sweat in clothes can enter the bodies of exchange friends (who typically exchange clothes). Through sweat they transfer *iware* and scent. Involuntarily, the sweat or other bodily substances of other persons can thus enter the body of a person bathing in the same water. Menstruating women therefore wash their sanitary cloths at low tide, well away from the village.[14] Poisons and invisible substances may enter the skin when they are actually directed at somebody else. The skin thus forms a crossroad of incoming and outgoing substances, which sometimes makes it hard to detect the origins of the revealed messages. A bad skin may be the result of internal as well as external pollution. Sufferers of a bad skin tend to point out external causes, whereas the people around them may be tempted to look for internal causes. Behavior and social relatedness are thus carefully analyzed. The identified source of pollution influences treatment choices.

Depending on the context, the skin forms a boundary between society and the individual, in which the individual is the external element, and between the individual and society, in which society is the external element. The skin further separates those with social connections and those without; those possessing *iware* and those without it; those showing morality and those who don't. It divides "flesh of one's own" from the bodies of nonrelated or nonassimilated people. Thus "society" or a "descent group" abstractly possesses a skin and a scent of its own, transcending individual boundaries. The skin also forms the boundary between life and death. Without a skin the body will rot and decompose. However, even this boundary is fluid, because flesh may start rotting before death.

The skin, finally, forms a boundary between generations: between mother and child, and old and young. It follows that if the boundaries disappeared, the oppositions between old and young, dead and alive, good and evil, the self and the other, fertility and infertility would disappear, and bodily substances would be shared completely. The skin therefore both provides a platform of social relations and facilitates them. Without borders between the self or the other, there would be no need for communication or exchange. We saw that these borders are fluid; depending on the context, they range from the individual body to society at large, and even include the land or the cosmos. These types of skin are often ascribed connotations similar to those of the human skin. The land can sweat (a reference to floods), for instance, or have a dry skin. Even treatment methods are comparable.

In summary, we have seen how on both the individual and the social level, different body parts are constructed or deconstructed, and function in relation to other bodies and other body parts. The flow of blood is, in Inanwatan, the central life-giving and life-taking system. It protects the core of the individual, the clan, or the society, and in this way ensures its maintenance. It accumulates and disposes of polluted substances in relation to other body substances and other bodies. Flesh embodies social relationships, whereas the skin reveals inner currents as well as external influences. Scent is the residue or resultant shared substance of these dynamics. To grasp the meaning and function of scent, we have defined its context within the boundaries of the individual body and of society at large. Scent has been related to the construction of flesh and to pollution of blood. Pollution, as a result of trespassing food and sexual taboos, has been indicated as the main cause of a foul scent, which is shed via the skin. Scent thus reveals morality, and divides people into people of the same scent and people of other scent, or people of one's own and the others, who may be (potential) *suangi*.

## THE SCENT OF TABOO, THE SCENT OF ILLNESS

Scent cannot be erased as easily as sweat; it gives a person away. Whereas the place or moment that sweat is shed can, to a certain extent, be controlled, scent is harder to hide. Scent sticks; it does not flow away as easily as sweat. It is possible to transfer scent to others through skin contact. In the following myth, in which several connotations of bodily exuviae are combined, we see an example of this. Scent is transported via sweat "out of place" (i.e., without the mediation of the skin), and via sexual contacts "out of place." There is no longer a boundary separating rotting substance from living matter, and sexual juices mix without restriction.

### The Story of Guri'ie

Once there was a man, Guri'ie was his name, from the *gobo* Kamenggo, they are the ones who have been decimated. This man had a fiancée who had died. But he had not been allowed to marry that girl, so she had married another man. She was called Garino. Garino had died, and her body was left behind on a platform. This Guri'ie, he was walking in the jungle, and discovered the corpse of that Garino. She was naked, she was left behind without covering or clothes, with her vagina uncovered, just like that. When he saw the girl like that, he wanted to have intercourse with her, although the body had died already two or three days ago. Guri'ie copulated with the girl until her skin burst open. She started to sweat, and she almost woke up again. Then this man wanted to go home, but he bathed first. The foul scent of the corpse stayed with him, its foul scent kept sticking on his body. He rubbed his body with leaves, but it did not help. In the end he went home, but in the village the people smelled that foul scent and asked who it was. It was Guri'ie, he was found out.

This girl had a husband, his name was Na'are. He went to check his wife in the graveyard. He looked at her and saw, Oh, her skin has already peeled off. He thought, Has somebody had sex with her, or what? He then looked at her vagina, and some sexual fluid came out. Na'are took a pearl shell and captured some of the sexual fluid in it. This he took home with him. When he came home, he cooked the fluid till it was boiling. Guri'ie went crazy, he frightened a lot of people. Guri'ie's father, Koria'e, embraced him because his child had gone mad, he wanted to break everything down. But he got out, he just disappeared. His father immediately went crazy himself, while his son had returned back to normal. Nobody could stop his father. Koria'e ran, he ran along the route used to go on a raid, and he gathered all the enemies. They returned to the village, led by that man. But his head just split like that, like a spirit, so nobody from his village could defeat him. Everybody was afraid of that spirit. That tribe then ran away until they met the Bobino people, who just finished them off.

Exchange, excretion, and handling of substances are present in a number of forms:

The naked skin and visible vagina of the dead Garino aroused illegal desire in Guri'ie.

Guri'ie spilled semen into the body of Garino without her consent.

Na'are collected the exuded fluid containing semen and vaginal fluid in a shell.

Fluid material is captured in an empty "skin" with a rough, wrinkled surface.

Na'are heats the fluid to cause an effect in the body of the excreter.

Intercourse and consequent intrusion of semen caused Garino's skin to burst and sweat.

Sweating and bursting skin are explained as caused by intercourse.

Garino's rotting flesh is revived directly through intercourse, or indirectly through sweating.

The foul scent of rotting flesh is transferred via this sweat to Guri'ie.

Bathing with water does not purify the skin.

The foul scent leads to identification by other people.

Through embracing (bodily or skin contact), illness (craziness, evilness) is transferred.

The patient is expelled (isolated) from the village.

The patient returns with a different identity (as a member of enemy group, or as "foreign").

Death makes the evil invisible (disembodied, face[head]less)

Invisible evil expels (decimates) society.

We see several expressions of substance "out of place," or individuals and groups "out of place," leading to illness and death, and order reversal. What started out as *iware* (semen and vaginal fluid) is transformed into infertility and death. A corpse comes to life, and a living body starts rotting. The sick become healthy, and the healthy become sick. Guardians of morality become embodied evil. Visible evil becomes invisible evil. Isolated evil isolates society. These reversals of order are mediated by the skin: naked skin caused desire "out of place," sweating skin caused revival, lack of skin caused transfer of the scent of rotting, coagulation in infertile skin (or empty core?) caused illness and death, skin contact caused transfer of traits, injured skin caused the escape of evil power, and vanished skin, finally, made this evil invisible and invincible.

This set of transformations is remarkably similar to perceptions of *suangi* and how it is transferred. It also reminds us of perceptions of sweating and skin diseases, and of some healing techniques that make use of sweat. Desire and greed have, in the previous sections, been associated with *suangi* and a foul-smelling sweat. A *suangi* steals blood and/or organs (i.e, skinless flesh) from its victims, and replaces them with *rotting* leaves. The process of rotting thus starts before death, or before decomposition of the skin. This causes a foul scent of the body (through sweating) and its excrement, which is described as black because it contains polluted blood. The skin of the victim is no longer solidly attached to its flesh; you can lift it up easily. This is a sign of weak flesh and bad skin.

A victim infected with *suangi* becomes a *suangi*. Once it is a *suangi*, the victim can transfer its powers to someone else without causing the death of that person. This is described as occurring through forced intercourse or strong embracing. A person may also look for *suangi* on his or her own initiative by consuming the corpse of a twin child, a child born to a woman defined as a *suangi*. A mother of twins is by definition *suangi:* she has stolen semen out of greed, thus possessing enough semen to produce two children instead of one. These various possibilities are thus based on consuming or absorbing substance out of place.

Killed *suangi* become *suangi* spirits, who are still capable of attacking people. That is why *suangi* are sometimes described as spirits instead of as living human beings. They can enter the body of an animal, thus disguising themselves. They change into—or enter the body of—a beautiful woman, and deceive or mislead their victims. Dead *suangi* victims similarly become *suangi* spirits. The evil force thus irrevocably infects others, and its power cannot be stopped. Previously, it is claimed, corpses of *suangi* were opened to look for proof; the presence of large quantities of dark blood (caused by eating rotting meat or rotting leaves) or double intestines are said to have given them away. Their bodies were then put in a canoe, which was released at low tide. In this way their corpses and their polluting essence were sent to the sea (isolated from the community). Alternatively, their bodies were put in a hollow tree trunk and burned. These methods are no longer applied because, informants said, this is not proper for Christians, and it is also impossible because of the presence of police and the army.

Nowadays a *suangi* is mainly fought with invisible counterweapons, such as prayer or sorcery. However, it is considered extremely difficult to destroy *suangi*. Invisibility, and a *suangi's* skill at deception, make it very hard to fight. *Suangi* is "out there," outside the moral community, but may physically be one of their own, destroying the community from the inside. Typically, a *suangi* attacks in-laws, but possibly also its own (nontwin) children. An informant described the threat of attack as follows:

> We no longer know who our enemies are, they use invisible forces. We are surrounded by evil, it is all around us. Sometimes I am afraid to go out, because I might be hit by something.

As *suangi* spreads, the moral community becomes smaller, and is finally encapsulated by it. The transformation has been completed. It is interesting to note that the spread of Christianity and extensive use of prayers have not, contrary to what might be expected from the stated use of prayer to counteract *suangi*, contributed to its destruction. Informants explain this by pointing out that these prayers are not used frequently enough by all members of the religious community—some merely fake their faith—or that these prayers are not the real sacral words that would do the job (the vicars keep those to themselves). Thus Christianity provided new moral weapons to counteract immoral attacks, but failed to distribute them equally among all members of society, which has led to an increase, rather than to a decline, of *suangi*.

What, then, would be the result of *suangi* attacks? They cause dysentery and chicken pox,[15] for instance, and severe bouts of malaria may also be caused by them. Water infected by a *suangi* corpse or spirit, or a *suangi* disguised as or sending mosquitoes who consume blood, infects the victims with malaria. Eating stolen food causes chicken pox. In both cases a patient sweats considerably and may die within a couple of days. Not infrequently, the question arises of why a particular person is infected, and others are not. The chances are that victims have (involuntarily) invited the attack by their behavior. If that is not the case, then these illnesses are perceived to be caused by accidentally consuming, encountering, or doing something that was actually intended for somebody else. These types of illnesses therefore always have a reason and are not explained as sheer coincidence, but leave room for claiming innocence. It is often claimed that formerly there was no dysentery or malaria. This could explain why these illnesses are only possible threats, whereas skin diseases leave no doubt about cause and guilt. Yaws and leprosy, for instance, are caused by self-chosen isolation, hoarding, or stealing. Flesh and skin have therefore started rotting before death, emanating a foul scent. Probably because their own bodies are affected, those with these diseases are regarded as less violent but nevertheless infective. Formerly, such patients were therefore left in the jungle to die or to cure themselves, after which they might return to society. They were thus isolated from society, and not attacked. Nowadays such practices no longer exist, but patients are still rather isolated and left to fend for themselves.

The foul scent of bodies released through the skin is thus the scent of rotting substances, substances that are "out of place" (because they are stolen or sent). Foul scent defines a person as immoral, as negating exchange of nurturing or nurtured substance. This has consequences for the way patients are treated and for their position within society. Their flesh is no longer the same; they have become different from other members of society. Before a person is defined as an outsider to the community, his or her behavior, grievances, relationships, enemies, and success are evaluated. Typically, in-married women, particularly those from other ethnolinguistic groups, and persons of low status are more prone to be suspected. Descendants of former slaves, for instance, have a lower status than descendants of former war heroes. People with a low status who have acquired wealth are suitable suspects, because they could have acquired their wealth through theft.

## PURIFICATION METHODS

Pollution of substances never stands alone, but is related to other substances or other bodies. Polluted blood, for instance, may be caused by a nurturing substance or an invisible poison, through intercourse or the possession of secret knowledge, or perhaps a spirit attack. It follows that healing methods take account of these different possibilities, and indeed a variety of methods are available. Sometimes the *ara'ugo* (soul) is traced and captured, or magical objects are pulled out of the skin, and perhaps an offering is made to ancestor spirits to restore the relationship with them. In most healing practices, water or smoke plays an important role. The skin is a significant route through which healing takes place. An *ara'ugo*, for instance, reenters the body through the skin. It is first captured in water. Fertility spells are uttered in water, sago, and tobacco, which have to be drunk, eaten, and smoked, respectively. The most secret part of the spell is uttered on the skin, through which the message is transported to the female womb. A trespasser of a major taboo is occasionally hidden behind smoke (i.e., his or her skin is made invisible and the scent is masked) to prevent spirit attack and consequent illness.

Purification is based on the excretion of the polluting substance, and this always occurs via the skin. Not surprisingly, the only possible cure for *suangi* attacks is excessive sweating. Attempts to cure such a victim follow a complicated pattern, because the cause of the ailment must first be defined. Once the ailment is diagnosed, the *suangi* is identified and negotiations to recover the *ara'ugo* begin. Only then is the sweating method applied. Finally, the identified *suangi* may be killed. The indigenous healer plays an important role in the entire process, but the sweat bath is undertaken in complete isolation to prevent infection. A patient usually tries a home remedy first, because the cause of the complaint is still unclear. Maybe it is just diarrhea, or "normal" malaria, or the blood is too weak for some other reason. Then food intake is altered to strengthen the blood. If this does not work, the patient and relatives start wondering if perhaps a spirit has attacked them, or somebody has sent an illness to them. *Suangi* is not the first cause to think about, unless there have been several attacks during the past couple of days.

A healer is called to the house of the patient. This usually takes place in late afternoon or when it is dark, because other people need not know what is going on. Healers are secretive about their healing capabilities; not everybody needs to know they possess them, because the capability to heal also implies the capability to send illness. They do not call themselves healers, and are not referred to as such; they are just "grandmothers who can read water" (*nenek yang mawe*) or "grandmothers who usually help us" (*nenek yang biasa bantu kita*). Healers therefore cure relatives first and foremost, rather than outsiders, and are slightly feared by the community. Patients also want to keep their illness as private as possible—in contrast to minor problems, such as nausea or wounds, for which sufferers claim a great deal of attention. Out of embarrassment, but also as a technique to surprise those who may have sent the illness, "real" illness is kept hidden as long as possible. The healer tries first to identify the illness by "reading" water (*mawe*). She locates the *ara'ugo* or *sombar,* because all more serious diseases involve soul loss in some way. Its location may tell her something about the cause. If the *ara'ugo* is roaming in the jungle, for instance, there may be a spirit involved, so the healer can proceed by negotiating with this spirit to retrieve the lost *ara'ugo.* The diagnosis is then soul loss, and the name of the illness depends on the spirit who has stolen it. In the case of *suangi*, however, it is extremely difficult to retrieve a soul because a *suangi* may already have consumed it. Even if the healer manages to retrieve it, the soul has likely been infected by *suangi* because it had been internalized within its body. The lost *ara'ugo* stays invisible in the water; the healer cannot "read" it, or can "read" it only with great effort. This leads to the first suspicions of *suangi*. If the patient also emanates a foul smell, this suspicion becomes stronger.

The healer identifies the *suangi* by looking once more into the water. This is the most feared part, because the healer might deceive her patient. Who knows if she manipulates the water, or tries to protect the *suangi*? In addition, the healer does not always reveal the identity of the *suangi* because she secretly wants to stage a counterattack. Calling out a name would attract the attention of the *suangi*, and even talking about *suangi* in general could inflict great harm.[16] Now that the healer knows the cause of the illness, she will try to negotiate with the *suangi* or attack it. She is believed to let her own *ara'ugo* travel to meet and fight the *suangi*, and then tries to retrieve the lost *ara'ugo*. If she succeeds, the *ara'ugo* enters the water, and this water is poured onto the patient, starting with the fontanelle; and smeared down to the shoulders, arms, and fingertips; then from the chest to the stomach; and finally from the upper legs to the toes. The healer "closes" the fontanelle, fingertips, and toes, so the *ara'ugo* will not leave again. The patient is urged to take steam baths to purify the body of the polluting, rotting substances inside it. These baths are taken in isolation, and the required medicinal leaves[17] have to be collected by the patient. The leaves are boiled in water. The pot is then placed within a tent made of mats woven from leaves, and the patient squats over it. The steam causes heavy perspiration. The steam and the tent hide the patient from the sight and smell of spirits, attracted by the scent of sweat, who could easily attack the vulnerable patient. Such an attack would make the illness even more complicated, but the covering should protect the patient sufficiently.

The mats are made out of leaves and play a role, for instance, in myths about floods; the causer of the flood is rolled in such a mat as protection against the wrath of spirits. These mats are also used to cover the dead and protect them against consumption by a corpse thief or *suangi*.[18] Concealment behind these mats during sweating thus perhaps not only functions to enhance sweating, but also to prevent further attacks by making the patient invisible and by suggesting the patient is already dead. The medicinal leaves are used to wipe off the excreted and polluted sweat, thus transferring the essence to the leaves. The remaining water is used to bathe the patient. Finally, the leaves are thrown into the ebbing tide, so they can leave the domain of the descent group, or they are thrown on a path:

> With the leaves you throw the illness away so someone else may step in it.

In this way the illness is not destroyed but transferred; somebody may tread on it or have contact with the water into which it was thrown. That someone else might die does not seem to bother anyone, because, they say, "We also got it from someone we may not even know."

It may, however, occur that the patient becomes more seriously ill, and it becomes hard to hide the illness from the outside world. The healer then claims that the *ara'ugo* has left again, and repeats her treatment. It may also happen that the *ara'ugo* of the *suangi* has entered instead, which requires exorcism. I have not witnessed such an exorcism because it hardly ever occurs, and is performed in private among a few relatives. From what I have heard, it may involve smoke (in a way similar to that used to hide trespassers of taboos). The heat and smoke drive the *suangi* out. It may also involve music, body decoration, and dance to cause trance in the healer, whose *ara'ugo* deceives the *suangi* with entertainment and desire for beautiful things such as gold. Then the distracted or incautious *suangi* can be attacked. How this occurs is not very clear. Some informants say the *suangi* is stabbed.[19] Older people say that the healer in fact sends the illness back, so the source dies by its own methods. There are not many healers left who are capable or willing to do that, because the chances are the healer will be attacked or infected by the *suangi*. Furthermore, they are reluctant to release its spirit, which could cause a larger threat for the community. The usual alternative is letting the patient die. A dead victim or a dead *suangi* cannot be buried in the same way as other people, or in the same location, because its contaminating juices pollute the soil. The patient has become a *suangi*, and there is hardly a way back. There is one more option left, and that is using steam baths. If a patient recovers, he or she will have beaten the *suangi*'s polluting essence, but it is never certain that the *suangi* possession is also cured. Such a patient remains vulnerable to accusations whenever somebody dies in a suspicious way. The cured patient may occasionally take on a new (secret) name and discard the old, unlucky one. The steam bath can, in that case, be seen as a temporary (mimicked) death and consequent rebirth to mislead the *suangi*.

The healing process is based on steps that involve identification of the illness through the scent of rotting, identification of the cause through the reading of water, isolation of the patient, publicly visible symptoms, purification of the soul through exorcism among related people, purification of the body through sweating in isolation, hiding or pretended death and reentry to society as a "new" person, disembodiment of the *suangi*, and consequent release of invisible danger that possibly threatens the entire society. This process follows, in general terms, the story of Guri'ie, or the coming and going of *suangi*. Indeed, a victim of attack is suspected to have invited it by greed or desire, and is treated accordingly. The victim is both subject and object, both the stage of the fight between "good" and "evil," or between Kekea'o and *suangi*, as well as the evil embodied. A cure disembodies this evil, moving the locality of the stage from skin to water, or from skin to soil. No wonder informants said that *suangi* has increased through time, and that there is no real cure for it. Purification externalizes and transfers the problem without really destroying it. Cured patients are therefore somehow responsible for illness in others; in being cured they are likely to infect others. Obviously this is an important reason why patients will not easily admit an attack and why there are no public healing rituals to cure patients and kill *suangi*.

For the sake of completeness, I should point out that patients often use a steam bath on their own initiative, without consulting a healer. They do this when they suspect someone has sent an illness to them, or when they only feel tired without a clear reason. Typically, this method is not applied when merely suffering from "plain" malaria, even though the symptoms may be the same as when *suangi* is suspected. When patients take a steam bath on their own initiative, this is not openly explained as *suangi*, but private suspicions are clearly involved. These baths are occasionally taken without the presence of any physical symptoms, but as a precaution—for instance, when a particular bird has flown over a person's house. This bird is called a *suangi* bird, and is one of the manifestations or disguises of *suangi*. Sometimes hanging certain leaves (see note 17) above the door is considered sufficient to ward off its evil influences. Another precaution is the planting of medicinal plants near the entrance and around the houses, which should ward off *suangi*. In one case neighbors of a man suspected of *suangi* had planted large amounts of ***daun suangi*** (*suangi* leaves) around their houses and had hung ***daun sukun*** near the windows and other openings in the house. Nobody had openly accused or attacked him. Their suspicions were fueled by his perceived self-chosen isolation and reluctance to share food, and some mentioned the number of his family members who had died.

Whereas at the beginning of my stay most people denied the existence of *suangi* in order to prevent accusations or attacks, it became central when, after a prolonged period of drought, many people suddenly became seriously ill and died. Speculations about the identity of the *suangi* followed, including some hunting expeditions by the adult men. They guarded the village by night to attack the *suangi*. Some claimed the *suangi* lived near the source domain, and ate the blood of the victims from a distance out of spite. Others said that the *suangi* lived in Inanwatan and owned land that his or her victims had entered illegally. Or was the *suangi* the spirit of a girl who had recently borne twins and died shortly afterward? Finally, some claimed the *suangi* was the thief who had lately been operating in the village and entered only the houses of people who hid money.[20] Most houses had leaves hanging above the entrance, and various families left the village to wait in their gardens until the *suangi* was caught.

When, weeks later, a dead *suangi* bird was found in the river, the hunt was finally declared successful. Its killing was never claimed publicly. The dead bird caused great anxiety; people stopped fishing, and looked or ran away. The water was taboo until the bird had drifted to the open sea. It was assumed that one of the healers had probably killed it in a magical fight, but did not want to make herself or the *suangi* known. The next person to die would have been the actual *suangi*. When an old man died whose nose was half gone due to "the bad disease" (or *tara bai*, a euphemism for leprosy and yaws), he was buried in silence. Nobody has talked about him since, nor has he been publicly accused.

He had become a taboo person. Once I asked why he had been singled out, and the only answer I got was that he had been greedy for money and made some women infertile. That was the last thing ever said about him. His name was not allowed to "stick" in memory. The source or medium of *suangi* had been expelled, but the question remained if indeed the bird had taken all its powers to the sea.

## THE ROTTING INTESTINES OF SOCIETY: SWEAT AND PURIFICATION OF THE SOCIAL BODY

Now that we have seen how purification of the body through sweating takes place, and what meanings are ascribed to foul-smelling sweat, we might wonder if this principle is also applied in a larger context, that of society. Earlier I claimed that certain processes taking place in society are compared to processes taking place in the body, such as rotting or the obstruction of the flow of blood, and that these are associated with increasing *suangi* and failing development. The perceived increase in *suangi* is described in terms of "the rotting of society" or "the consumption of the intestines of society" and "weakened flesh and blood." It is explained by the loss of secret knowledge (*iware*), by greed for personal gain, by too liberal sexual relations, or by increased distance from the source domain and disturbance of the relationship with the ancestors (the core, "bones"). Loss of knowledge and the latter two reasons are related to the increased influence of Christianity, and the church's apparent lack of proper replacements or willingness to share them. The increase in *suangi* is thus primarily associated with the loss of indigenous values or morals without proper replacements, and with body substances out of place. The only way to destroy it, on this level, is through a major counteract by God or Kekea'o herself. One (female) informant described the nearing end as follows:

> God comes in many disguises, mostly covered by a bad skin, in a bad body. He lives in a very small and shabby house, and he will save those who live like him. You have to treat him well and give him food, so he will reveal himself to you and say "I know you, do you know me?" I have seen him lately, for instance, in Sorong. He had put on a really bad skin, with a skin disease, and his body smelled bad. He asked someone for food, but she refused initially because he smelled revolting. Finally she gave him really bad food, just the remnants, on dirty dishes, and while he was eating, the tears came pouring down his cheeks. When he had finished, he thanked her for the food and said that he now knew her. Her whole family dropped dead instantly. I saw him after that happened. Now he was a handsome young man asking me for money to buy a piece of cloth. I went with him to the shop where he wanted to buy it, but he did not have enough money. The shopkeeper did not want to lower his very high price, so I helped him with my money. He told me about the nearing test. He then burned the shop down with his eyes. The end is near now, but only those who know when will survive. You have to prepare enough food and remain indoors when the flood comes. When the flood is gone, there will be a drought, and many people will die of hunger or burn in the flames. Then the

world will flip over, and those living below will come up. We will finally be reunited with our ancestors.

This reminds us of Darrouzet's comments on the relationship between sorcery, purification, and millenarian wishes in the Bogia district of Papua New Guinea:

> . . . milleniarism promises, among other things, transcendence of death. For primitive consciousness, which understands sorcery and related phenomena to be at the root of all death, transcendence of death requires that sorcery itself be transcended one way or the other. (1985:78–79)

Stewart and Strathern inferred from Darrouzet's comments on sorcery and development that

> people expressed their concern about the problem of sorcery generally and their wish to eradicate it as a practice, i.e. to purify the new politico-economic space of their existence in order to obtain the benefits of "development." (1997a:20; see Darrouzet 1985:105)

The relationship between overcoming evil and development opportunities is certainly present in Inanwatan, where God will initiate the end of the present world order in order to separate "good" from "evil," and restore the cosmic order by breaking the boundaries of body and cosmos. Related to the above observations on sorcery and development, Stewart and Strathern conclude that

> one of the common themes that run through many of the narratives of assault sorcery [which definition closely resembles *suangi*, see Stewart and Strathern 1997a:6] is that of breaching the body to perpetuate destruction. . . . These actions of assault sorcery are in many aspects the antithesis of aspects of fertility ritual. (1997a:21)

Similarly, in Inanwatan a flood will break all boundaries and destroy all life. The water (sweat) comes from inside the earth, boiling up through openings in the land. The surface of the earth (skin) will be covered with water, and will swallow most lives. The flood is thus poured through the "skin," and the dirt from the "flesh" and "blood" (i.e., the immoral conduct of people), travels with it. The emerging foul scent is explained as coming from the decaying corpses and the "rotting flesh of society."

Those possessing true faith in God will be able to escape death by staying indoors and preparing sufficient supplies of food to survive until the water level drops again. This vision is remarkably similar to the practice of steam baths in which the dirt comes out along with the sweat, and patients hide themselves. What is perhaps even more interesting is that survival is considered possible only if people behave like a *suangi* by isolating themselves and hoarding food, though in reality they do this because God has instructed them. It seems to me that what we have here is a reversal of roles or purposeful "identity confusion"; by ***disguising*** themselves as *suangi,* the water will not be able to capture them, just as a healer cannot capture a stolen soul in her bowl of water. The question remains where the polluted residue is left, and so far no uniform answer has been given. On the one hand, this is no longer relevant because *iware* is restored and flows fluently again, but on the other hand, some do envision a prolonged period of drought and consequent hunger and fires, which will "finish the job." Again only those who have hoarded food and drinking water and stay inside will survive, whereas those who have to go out to look for food will be consumed by the fire. The fire (smoke) will not be able to reach and destroy those who stay indoors, just as smoke is used to hide a patient. *Suangi* is thus destroyed by disguise, by *acting like one.*

In a similar way, those who had survived a great flood that occurred in the mythical past warded off the water by staying inside their house in the jungle. Others refused to help aged relatives, and yet others killed a hunting dog. Self-isolation, refusal to take care of dependent relatives, and killing and wasting an important food source—acts that under normal circumstances would be despised saved their lives. In this context, acting in an immoral manner is defined as temporarily acceptable by a moral agency, be it the ancestors or God. The real *suangi* will be revealed and destroyed by flowing water and (active) fire, as opposed to revelation and healing by *heated* (passive) substance or *contained* water. This is surprisingly reminiscent of what Stewart and Strathern wrote about sorcery in Papua New Guinea and Australia: "The concealment and revelation aspects of assault sorcery *mirror* those of other ritual dramas" (1997a:21; emphasis added). Being an antithesis or mirror of healing rituals, however, *suangi* is in turn destroyed by deception and disclosure—in short, by application of its own tactics.

The idea of mimicking or deception is, in Inanwatan, also present in opposite forms. The favorite disguise of God, for instance, is a repulsive old beggar, whereas those who disguise themselves as innocent and social persons, which is exactly what *suangi* are believed to do, die. This wider context of *suangi* destruction, finally, helps to explain some of the anxiety involved in individual attacks. Because treatment largely follows the way people are infected with *suangi*, we could argue that by mimicking such an attack, the *suangi* will be counteracted or even fooled (confused by the false identity of the victim) and try to find another victim. At the same time, however, other people can never be sure if this deception or counteraction has indeed worked. It does not guarantee that the attacker has been destroyed, not just distracted for the time being. The skin may not always reveal the hidden dimension. The only signal that cannot be mimicked is, of course, scent. The foul scent of sweat ultimately gives the real *suangi* away.

This intriguing mixture of deception and counterdeception makes it clear to us that things, in Inanwatan, are not always what they seem. This could even be said of the suggestion of possession of *iware*, on the one hand, and the protection and enclosure of it, on the other. Or, for that matter, of the overt discarding of practices and beliefs (such as the public burning of harmful spells or claiming that *suangi* no longer exists), and their continuation in different forms or localities. The church has also been the object of notions of deception and counterdeception, and evaluated as either a way to salvation that is open to those who really understand and sincerely follow its teachings, or as a disguised evil that has penetrated to the heart of Inanwatan society, destroying the moral community from the inside.

The only way to really know the truth is through scent. When, in Inanwatan, people say that all Inanwatan smell the same and share the same flesh and blood, they are actually making a moral statement. Those who are greedy must smell bad, and those who smell bad must be greedy. Scent is therefore not just an objective or individual experience, but collectively and morally encoded. In the context of health and healing, it defines both morality and identity: Is someone victim or cause, of the same or different flesh and blood? Scent is therefore more than just a bodily excretion; it is a watershed between the self and the other, or between the moral community and the world beyond.

## NOTES

1. Interestingly, immigrants living in the area found the body odor of the local population repellent, and vice versa. As a newcomer I noticed a difference in body odor between the Inanwatan population and the other Indonesians. The local Inanwatan initially smelled sourer and more penetrating than I was used to. I thought at that time that it was perhaps caused by differences in food, and the Inanwatan population claimed that this was indeed an important aspect.

2. This process has been defined by A. Strathern for the New Guinea Highlands as a "grease cycle" (1982:118).

3. From examples in other parts of New Guinea, it is clear that this notion of a closed or bounded system is quite widespread. The southern "fringe" groups such as the Etoro and the Bedamini, for example, have a similar point of view (see Marx 1994:36, 39).

4. In another context informants said that Kekea'o was in fact God, who is described as a very old and wrinkled man.

5. This term is rather widespread in parts of eastern Indonesia, including the Bird's Head and the Moluccas.

6. Compare this to M. Strathern's description of the Melanesian body: "The body, then, has no inherent properties or capacities . . . the body features as a register, a site of . . . interaction. . . . It is a microcosm of *relations*" (1988:131).

7. This is rather common in other parts of Melanesia as well. In Fiji, for instance, weight loss and thinness are associated with "social neglect or deprivation" (Becker 1995:38).

8. We find a striking similarity to Fijian associations between sharing food and morality: "The community's moral qualities are symbolically condensed in bodies, which record and reflect the care vested in them" (Becker 1995:85).

9. Not surprisingly, this also applies to yams in the Dobuan context: "Consuming one's own yams becomes a metaphor for consuming one's own sisters. What

we seem to have here then, is the symbolic equation between cannibalism and incest" (Bloch and Parry 1982:28).

10. Presently such initiation practices are a mere shadow of what they are claimed to have been. Some elder men said they still secretly initiate boys, suggesting that there probably are still some men who practice it.

11. Because their husbands contained their uncles' semen, women had to avoid the uncles to prevent suggestions of adultery.

12. See also A. Strathern: "The skin, the outer self, is the immediate point of contact with the physical world outside them and can also conveniently symbolise the point of contact between themselves and the social forces that surround them" (1977:101).

13. O'Hanlon likewise saw such a relationship for the decorated skin: "The quality of the decorated appearance and the inner moral state of those involved are felt to reflect each other" (1989:138).

14. The life force or polluting residues of those living at the source of the river is thus transported to settlements downstream, and the residues of those living in the river mound can be transported to those living upstream at high tide. This has implications for settlement patterns.

15. I do not have sufficient medical training to judge whether the symptoms were of these diseases. During an outbreak of *suangi*, medical staff from the Health Centre defined the symptoms as dysentery.

16. It therefore was several months before informants wanted to talk about *suangi*. It could even cause accusations.

17. These contain *daun suangi (suangi* leaves, which are usually planted around the house as protection), *daun kelor* (leaves used to make a protective fence around the house), and *daun sukun* (leaves used to ward off spirits). These types of plants are all used to defend a house against illnesses and intruders.

18. Recall that Garino was laid out naked and unprotected, and thus attracted the desire of Guri'ie.

19. In myth Kekea'o destroys a *suangi* by burning her, and another one by splitting her head. This reminds us of the way the evil father of Guri'ie was killed. Perhaps the healer reenacts the way Kekea'o defeated *suangi*.

20. These were the houses of people responsible for the collection or division of funds to improve the standard of living in the village. The kiosks, where probably more money or goods were stored, were strangely enough left untouched.

## REFERENCES

Becker, A. E. 1995. *Body, Self, and Society: The View from Fiji*. Philadelphia: University of Pennsylvania Press.

Bloch, M., and J. Parry. 1982. Introduction: Death and the regeneration of life. In M. Bloch and J. Parry, eds., *Death and the regeneration of life*, pp. 1–44. Cambridge and London: Cambridge University Press.

Darrouzet, C. 1985. *Sorcery, Salvation, and the Politics of Death in a Lowland New Guinea Society: A Case Study of a Modernizing Culture and Consciousness*. Ann Arbor, MI: University Microfilms International.

Elmberg, J.E. 1968. *Aspects of Tradition and Change Among the Mejprat of the Ajamaru District of the Bird's Head (Vogelkop).* Monograph Series, Publication no. 12. Stockholm: Ethnographic Museum.

Goldman, L.R. 1995. The depths of deception: Cultural schemas of illusion in Huli. In A. Biersack, ed., *Papuan Borderlands: Huli, Duna, and Ipili Perspectives on the Papua New Guinea Highlands,* pp. 111–140. Ann Arbor: The University of Michigan Press.

Haga, A. 1884. *Nederlands Nieuw-Guinea en de Papoese Eilanden: Historische Bijdrage, 1500–1883.* 2 vols. Batavia, Java: W. Bruinig; The Hague: Martinus Nijhoff.

Kahn, M. 1986. *Always Hungry, Never Greedy: Food and the Expression of Gender in a Melanesian Society.* Cambridge: Cambridge University Press.

Loudon, J.B. 1977. On body products. In J. Blacking, ed., *The Anthropology of the Body,* pp. 161–178. London, New York: Academic Press.

Marx, K. 1994. *Blood, Semen, and Fears: Body Substance Ideologies and Gender in New Guinea.* Ann Arbor, MI: U.M.I. Dissertation Services.

O'Hanlon, M. 1989. *Reading the Skin: Adornment, Display and Society Among the Wahgi.* London: British Museum Publications.

Stewart, P. J., and A. J. Strathern. 1997a. *Sorcery and Sickness: Spatial and Temporal Movements in Papua New Guinea and Australia.* Discussion Paper Series no. 1. Centre for Pacific Studies, James Cook University of North Queensland.

Stewart, P. J., and A. J. Strathern. 1997b. *Transecting Bisects: Female Spirit Cults as a Prism of Cultural Performance in the Hagen, Pangia, and Duna Areas of Papua New Guinea.* Okari Research Group Working Paper no. 1. Pittsburgh: Department of Anthropology, University of Pittsburgh.

Strathern, A. J. 1977. Why is shame on the skin? In J. Blacking, ed., *The Anthropology of the Body,* pp. 99–110. London and New York: Academic Press.

Strathern, A. J. 1982. Witchcraft, greed, cannibalism and death: Some related themes from the New Guinea Highlands. In M. Bloch and J. Parry, eds., *Death and the Regeneration of Life,* pp. 111–133. Cambridge: Cambridge University Press.

Strathern, M. 1988. *The Gender of the Gift.* Berkeley: University of California Press.

# CHAPTER 3

# The Manes Kaya Healing Rite: Blood, Sago, and Sacred Cloths for the Ancestors

*Ien Courtens*

Every weekday morning, inhabitants of the village of Ayawasi, in west Ayfat, Irian Jaya, assemble in front of the missionary outpatient clinic. At eight o'clock precisely, one of the nurses opens the door to the waiting room and the patients enter. Slowly, they take a seat on the wooden benches along the wall, and wait patiently for the nurse to hand them a number. Most days the room is crowded immediately, filled with up to eighty men, women, and children.

Thus, in present-day Ayfat society,[1] located in the interior of the Bird's Head of Irian Jaya, it seems clear that Western notions of illness and curing have grown important. During my fieldwork I noticed that the majority of the people who get ill usually initially visit the outpatient clinic.[2] The clinic in Ayawasi was founded in 1963 by the Dutch Missionary Sisters of the Precious Blood (CPS). Some years later the sisters also established a little laboratory. Through the years, the services of the hospital became increasingly important for inhabitants of Ayawasi and surrounding villages.

Before the introduction of Catholicism, female and male healers practiced indigenous healing methods. They gained their spiritual knowledge of healing during initiation rites. In addition, many women received knowledge about healing through dreams in which ancestral spirits revealed the methods to apply. Within the local missionary process indigenous healing practices have altered and new ways of healing have emerged. Nevertheless, I soon discovered that, simultaneously, various forms of indigenous healing practices remain important and that indigenous conceptions about illness and healing play a central role in daily life. Initiated men are still respected ritual specialists. Women rely on the spiritual knowledge of healing they gain through dreams and clan-bound healing rituals are still common practice. I came to see that in the Ayfat area, as in other parts of the Pacific region (Baddeley 1985; Macpherson 1985; Stephen 1987; Trompf 1991), people nowadays divide illness into two categories. Those categories are not perceived by local peoples as conflicting, but rather as complementary. The first, which includes malaria and influenza, is seen as a biological reaction of the body: as illness due to a natural cause, such as a mosquito bite or a cold caught while walking in the rain. For treatment people frequently visit the hospital, and Western medical treatment is highly appreciated.

The second type of illness can be classified as part of the indigenous religious belief system, for instance, illness as a form of ancestral punishment, sorcery (caused by initiated men), or witchcraft (caused by female witches). Illness as a form of ancestral punishment takes an especially important place in present-day Ayfat communities.

This chapter concerns the latter type of illness. It examines the Manes Kaya rite,[3] an indigenous rite that is performed to heal persons who have been made ill by ancestral spirits. Although "spirit illness" is seen all over the Pacific islands (Courtens 1998; Haiveta 1990; Keck 1992; Mageo and Howard 1996; Mitchell 1990; Parsons 1985; Schieffelin 1996), cause and treatment may vary by region. In the case presented here, the ritual is performed to cure a middle-aged man who was punished by the spirits of his ancestors because he had violated ancestral laws. In this ritual, I explore healing in terms of spiritual and kinship relations. In doing so, I agree with Keck (1992:326), who argues that in Pacific societies, "illness is closely connected with social and kin-group relations and can only be explained in terms of their belief system."

During the performance of the Manes Kaya ritual, one kind of humor, blood, is especially important. In northwest Ayfat, blood is a central notion not only with regard to social relations (Schoorl 1979:130; Miedema 1984:135) but also with regard to illness and health. Illness is usually refered to as "having dirty blood" (***darah kotor***) or "having less blood" (***kurang darah***). Illness occurs when the correct balance of the blood is disrupted. Only by restoring the balance, by means of a healing rite, a person can be cured. The imbalance of the blood is represented in conditions of "hot" and "cold." Because illness is associated with a "hot" state, the aim of the ritual is to "cool down" the patient, that is to "clean the dirty blood" or to "increase the blood." The central symbolic meaning of blood is also expressed in various ways during the Manes Kaya rite, in which the blood of a pig is crucial. Simultaneously, the vital organs of a pig (the heart, liver, and lungs), sacred cloths, and sago are central symbols that are offered to the ancestors while inviting them "to come down" to cure the sick person.

In daily and ceremonial life throughout the Bird's Head area of Irian Jaya, cloths (***kain timur***) play a central role. Although these cloths have been imported centuries ago from east Indonesia, they are generally referred to as "indigenous" by native people. Moreover, the cloths have been incorporated to such a great extent in daily and ceremonial life that they are central in ancestor worship, because the sacred cloths (***kain pusaka***) are believed to be connected to the ancestors.[4]

The performance of the Manes Kaya rite, in which I participated during my fieldwork, will be described and analyzed. I will focus on blood, as the central humor, in relation to the other significant symbols of food and sacred cloths. The major aim of this chapter is to explore relationships between these central symbols and notions of sickness and health. In particular, I will focus on the curative and protective characteristics of blood in the Manes Kaya rite.[5]

Following Laderman and Roseman (1996:2), I will approach the Manes Kaya healing rite as a cultural performance, ". . . fusing past traditions and memories with present circumstances and problems." Consequently, emphasis will be on the performance as an active event. Before I describe the healing rite, I will turn briefly to indigenous beliefs about spirits in northwest Ayfat.

## SPIRITS

Throughout the northwest Ayfat area, maintaining a good relation with ancestral spirits is a necessary condition for prosperity in life. Transgression of ancestral laws is immediately punished by the spirits through severe illness or misfortune. Despite the fact that they risk adversity, descendants regularly do not comply with the rules, mostly out of negligence.

According to indigenous notions, spirits of deceased persons reside in *seweron*,[6] which is located underground and nowadays is equated with the Christian heaven. From there the spirits watch over and protect their relatives. As elsewhere, however, it is common for spirits to visit the world of the living. Generally, they meet at night. Spirits can manifest themselves in dreams that convey messages to their descendants. Knowledge about healing is often gained through dreams in which ancestral spirits reveal the methods to apply. Messages can also contain a warning of danger or advice on major decisions concerning clan or personal affairs. In return for protection and advice, the spirits of the ancestors expect obedience and respect from their kin. People generally honor their ancestors by offering cigarettes and food (either with or without matches, spoon, and fork) on their graves.

Spirits can do more than reveal themselves in dreams. After sunset, they can leave *seweron* and wander around the village, knocking on people's doors or making scary noises. By doing so, the spirits haunt or frighten a person who has exceeded or disregarded ancestral rules. Once in the village, spirits can also discipline the descendants by taking possession of a person's body, thus making someone seriously ill.

On the other hand, ancestral spirits have the power to cure. In case the illness is caused by ancestral spirits, people can choose particular indigenous healing rites. One of the possibilities is to consult male or female indigenous healers, who generally perform by means of herbal therapies. Sometimes the illness requires a more extensive healing ritual. If such is the case, a clan-bound indigenous healing rite, such as Manes Kaya, can be performed. The aim of the ritual is to worship the ancestors and to request their help for recovery, to restore the balance of the blood.

In the Ayfat region, every extended family group has its own clan-bound healing rite. Usually the rites have different names, yet the proceedings are more or less the same. A healing ritual such as Manes Kaya generally takes place in a food garden, away from the village, and is accessible only to people who belong to the same clan. In this case the sick person belongs to the clan Baru, and therefore only people who share common ancestors with the Baru attend the healing performance. Not only are people with the same ancestors allowed to participate in the healing ritual, they are obliged to participate for the sake of pleasing the ancestors. If they do not participate, the ancestors will punish them, and consequently they will be taken ill.

## A CLAN-BOUND HEALING RITUAL

Agus Baru, a man in his late fifties, lives in a small village in north Ayfat. One day Agus falls very ill. It starts with a minor stomach ache, but soon the pain increases. He loses a lot of weight, can hardly eat anything, and has a high fever. First, Agus consults Matius Titit, a male relative who is a well-known indigenous healer in his home town. He gained spiritual knowledge of healing during initiation rites in the *wuon* cult house. Matius treats Agus by means of herbal therapy. As is customary with these symptoms, Matius prepares the vigorously active root *bofiet*. For one week, Agus has to take drops of the sap.[7] The treatment, however, is ineffective: Agus's condition deteriorates.

In his search for a cure, Agus decides to visit his sister Maria Baru in the village of Ayawasi in west Ayfat, and to seek medical treatment in the missionary hospital there. After he has been hospitalized for almost three months there still is no recovery. Maria can no longer stand by and watch Agus's worrying state of health. Maria is a well-known and respectable healer. She learned about indigenous healing when she was a novice in the female initiation rite *fenia meroh*, in the 1960s. In the 1980s, after she experienced Christian visions in which God revealed himself and sent her divine messages on the application of Christian healing, Maria Baru became the founder and leader of a special Christian prayer group (Courtens 1998). Members of the group, who all experienced visions, reside throughout the Bird's Head and act as ritual healers. As a ritual specialist within the prayer group, Maria combines Christian symbols, such as the crucifix, a statuette of the Virgin Mary, a rosary, and holy water, with indigenous healing notions and practices, like dreaming or the application and bespelling of medicinal leaves, roots, and tree bark. Besides Christian visions, Maria Baru has received ancestral messages, in which her deceased parents gave her the necessary strength and power to act as a healer, and instructed her in different ways of indigenous healing. Especially when the illness is caused by ancestral spirits, Maria Baru will perform an indigenous healing rite, such as the Manes Kaya rite.

According to indigenous religious notions, if Western treatment is ineffective, the illness is most likely caused by interference of ancestral spirits. So, for the sake of curing her brother Agus, Maria turns to her ancestors and requests their help. That night Maria has a vivid dream. She sees images of many sacred cloths and a dead pig. The next morning Maria confronts her brother with the dream. Suddenly, Agus recalls a significant event that happened some months ago. At that time, he did not think it was important, but now, because he is seriously ill, Agus realizes that he did not obey a particular ancestral rule. Cautiously, he tells his story. One day, Petrus Titit, a male relative, asked Agus to lend him one of the clan's sacred cloths. Petrus needed the cloth for a major rite. Agus, as one of the clan elders, wanted to fulfill his social and kin-group obligations, so he gave the cloth on loan. In time, Petrus returned the cloth to Agus. Agus then handed the woven fabric over to his sister Aknes, who stored the cloth in a safe place.[8]

At first sight, there seems nothing wrong with the procedure. Nevertheless, Agus omitted to hold a ceremony to assure his ancestors that the cloth had returned safely. Agus now realizes that, for disregarding the rule, he is punished by his ancestors, who are upset by his behavior. Only a clan-bound ritual can redeem his mistakes. Thus, Maria decides to perform the Manes Kaya healing rite in one of her food gardens to worship the ancestors. By her doing so, Agus is given the opportunity to ask forgiveness of the spirits and to reconcile the disturbed relationship with the ancestors.

## Sacred Cloths

The food garden is just outside the village. A small path that leads to it twists through the woods. Ferns grow on either side, under the tall trees that enclose the village. At one point a little stream interrupts the muddy track. A wooden fence surrounds the food garden to prevent wild pigs from entering and eating the crops. High cassava plants overgrow the place.

Earlier that day, at sunrise, Maria Baru and Matius Titit, who accompanied Agus to Ayawasi, had gone to the food garden to make the necessary preparations. They built two bamboo platforms, one higher than the other, on the empty space in front of the little pile dwelling close to the entrance of the food garden.

It is late in the afternoon when everyone gathers in the garden. Some men put the final touches to the lower platform. With a liana they tie the bamboo sticks. A pile of leaves, *daun rotan*, lies ready for the sago to be bundled. Children run around with each other, or sit patiently with the adults on the little wooden ladder or on the small porch of the garden house, waiting for the healing rite to start.

Maria checks to see if everything is in order. She takes her carrying bag, *eyu*, and removes an *am* (woven mat) from it. The *am* is filled with *kain timur*, six pieces in total. She unfolds the mat on the ground in front of her, and one by one she displays the cloths on the woven mat. Five cloths, which are named *wan Fas, pokek Safah, wan Ataf, wan Habeh, and wan Warnau*, are very old and carefully wrapped in little packages made of leaves (*daun koba*). The colors have faded, and the cloths are here and there stitched with little pieces of textile. The sixth cloth is new fabric, wrapped in plastic, and is called Batik Irian.

The sick man, Agus Baru watches his younger sister from the garden house. Slowly he steps down and arranges the sacred cloths on the mat. "We have to speak clearly and slowly, otherwise the spirits of our ancestors cannot hear us well," Agus explains to his relatives. Then Agus looks up in the air and invokes his ancestors: "Look at us. We are making everything ready for you, here, in our food garden, on your territory."

In the meantime Maria fetches the pig, which she will sacrifice especially for this occasion, from under the garden house. Arit Baru, the younger brother of Agus and Maria's deceased father, steps forward. He is the first to take one of the sacred cloths, and holds it in front of him, his arms stretched above his head. While he focuses his eyes on the *kain timur*, he addresses his ancestors and shouts: "I open this sacred cloth to show you that everything here is all right." Matius joins Agus. Together they unfold the second cloth. Agus gets up to speak, and explains to the ancestral spirits:

> I give this festive meal [*pesta makan*] together with my clan members, both schoolchildren and adults, because I'm ill. Because I did not listen to you, because I did not obey your laws. I did not arrange to give a ceremony before, as I promised our ancestor Pofitsteyuo, to show you that this sacred cloth returned to our clan.[9]

This act marks a crucial moment in the healing rite. By opening the sacred cloth, Agus fulfills one of his ceremonial obligations. The showing of sacred cloths to the ancestors is central in every major indigenous rite. It is done not only during healing rituals but also, for instance, during funerals of local leaders or other prominent men and women.

The ritual continues. Simultaneously, the three men start reciting the names of their ancestors.[10] Sometimes the men stop for a moment before resuming their recitation of the long list of names. Agus continues his speech: "Within a minute, I will kill a pig, bundle sago, and give back to you your sacred cloth." Maria adds: "Now this sacred cloth is back in our family again." The rest of the cloths are unfolded while Agus tells his ancestors that the sacred cloths are kept safe within his family.

> Do not think we gave these cloths away, brought them to other places. But I am ill. My stomach aches. I vomit, have diarrhea, high fever. I know you are angry with me. You have made me ill. You are in my stomach, because I did not listen. But now I give this festive meal and return to you this *kain pusaka*.

In turn Arit, Matius, and Maria emphasize Agus's words by explaining to the spirits that Agus is very ill: "He almost died, and even the sisters of the missionary hospital could not find a way to cure him." Then Agus invites his ancestors:

Maria will sacrifice this pig for you. We will offer you sago. Come and eat with us. Then leave. Go home, back to your mountain,[11] and do not come back. Do not disturb us again. Make us strong, so we can work in our food gardens and have a good harvest. Do not let a wild pig enter the food garden and eat all the crops. Now the sacrifice can start. I am ready.

Next, another crucial part of the ritual is performed, in which the ties with the ancestors who caused Agus's illness will be broken off.

## Blood

The cloths, except the Batik Irian, are draped over a branch of a young tree that grows next to the higher platform. A cord is attached to the top of the tree. The tree represents Agus, the sick person. The cord symbolizes the spirits of their ancestors. Maria takes the cord in one hand while in her other hand she holds a string that is tied to one of the pig's feet. For the last time the four relatives invoke their ancestors together by calling out their names.

Agus takes the sacred cloth *wan Fas* from the branch, puts it on the pig's back before he shouts: "Kill the pig!" Maria still holds the cord that leads to the tree with the *kain timur*. She is next to Agus, and hands him the string tied to the pig. They join their free hands.

One of the younger men, Marcellino Hay, lifts a big stick with his two hands. With a harsh blow the branch falls upon the pig's head. The animal collapses, squealing loudly. Simultaneously, Matius severs the cord attached to the young tree, symbolically severing the ties with the spirits who made Agus ill (as Maria Baru explained to me later).

Agus watches Marcellino strike the skull of the pig a few more times. When blood runs out of the pig's nostrils, Agus bends over. At this point in the ritual, the central meaning of blood comes to the fore. With a righthand finger Agus strokes through the bright red blood, then rubs the blood on his chest, in the middle of his breastbone. Everyone watches with bated breath, because it is an important moment in the ceremony. With his shirt unbuttoned, Agus shows his token to the onlookers. With this blood mark Agus makes clear to his ancestors that he sacrificed a pig especially for them. He then begs his ancestors:

Do not eat me again. Come down and eat this pig, which we will cook for you. In exchange, "close" my stomach, give me back my health. Pofitsteyuo, do not ever again say that I did not listen to you. This festive meal is especially for you and for all my ancestors. Come down and take everything we offer you.

In case the illness is caused by spirits, in northwest Ayfat people usually explain their illness as being "eaten up" by these spirits. Sometimes people say that spirits are "in" their body. Therefore, food is offered to invite the ancestors to come and eat the food instead. Sacrifice is the highest honor that can be given to the worshiped ancestors. Therefore, the best of all is offered: a pig, and especially, its vital organs. The sacrificial death indicates the importance of this animal: a pig is considered worth offering to the spirits. As is seen throughout New Guinea, illness that has not responded to other treatments requires the slaughter of a pig. To convince Agus's ancestors that a pig is offered, a blood mark is applied to his body. On the one hand, the blood mark on Agus's chest (or any other sick part) is proof that a pig is sacrified. On the other hand, the sign will simultaneously safeguard Agus, "close" his body and prevent the spirits from "entering" and "eating" him again. By sacrificing a pig for the spirits of the ancestors, Agus exchanges the animal for recovery of his health. In this way, blood has the capacity to heal and protect.

In the meantime, the pig still lies on the ground, half conscious, its stomach moving quickly in rhythm with its breathing. Some young men make a fire from a large pile of branches and leaves. When the fire blazes up brightly, they throw the pig in the flames. With a final effort the animal offers resistance and jumps out of the flames. Immediately it is thrown back. More wood is put on the fire, and quickens the death of the pig.

## Sago

While the young men are occupied with roasting the pig, Maria spreads another *am* just before the higher platform, in front of the garden house. "Now let us bundle the sago we all brought with us and prepared for this festive dinner, to present to our ancestors," she says.

Like most rituals in Melanesia, the *Manes Kaya* ritual is closely bound up with food. Not only does the family sacrifice a pig, they also offer sago to the ancestors. Sago is supposed to come from the land belonging to the ancestors, which the clan members inherit from generation to generation. Futhermore, sago forms a substantial means of existence. In case the food gardens yield light crops, people can always rely on their sago fields.

Then, from the narrow porch of the garden house, Maria lifts a big pan filled with sago porridge. She spreads the sago on leaves *(daun rotan)* she has laid out on the woven mat. She folds up the stuffed leaves, winds a liana around them, and piles the long, narrow bundles next to her. Arit, who has taken a seat on the higher platform, assists Maria by handing her the lianas. Maria's daughter Yosefin, and Matius kneel on the mat to help Maria bundle the sago. Agus sits on top of the garden house ladder, exhausted.

While the pig roasts in the fire, the young men scrape the scorched hair from its skin with a big chopping knife (*parang*). After some twenty minutes, they take the pig out of the fire and lay it on its back, before the lower platform.

They open it from both sides of the snout down along the flanks. Dogs lick the blood from the mouth of the blackened animal.

Then Agus comes down the ladder. Taking some sago in one hand and rattan leaves in the other, he invokes the ancestors for the last time:

Spirits, please eat this food I offer you. You have to eat this and then leave, go home. The food, the meat and the *kain timur* I already gave back to you . . . everything is for you. My clan members and I, together we give you all this.

Arit, Matius, and Maria complete Agus's plea for help by asking the ancestors "to leave Agus" and "to leave Ayawasi." Because they have now fulfilled their ancestral obligations, the spirits have no reason anymore to be angry over Agus's behavior. Simultaneously, they ask their ancestors to watch over the clan members: "Keep us and our children safe. Keep us healthy and let our food gardens bear a rich harvest."

Some time later, they finish the sago bundles. Carefully, Maria and Yosefin carry the stuffed leaves to the lower platform, where they spread the bundles next to each other. The packages cover the platform. Maria then covers up the bundles with the rest of the *daun rotan*.

A young boy wipes clean the bamboo canes that stood against one of the trees. Children bring them to the men cutting the pig, while women lay out vegetables (*sayur pakis*). Maria squats down, takes a bamboo cane, and fills the hollow tube with hunks of meat and vegetables. Meanwhile, one of the girls chops new canes from long bamboo stalks. One by one, Maria stuffs the sixty-centimeter-long canes.

**Ancestors**

The ritual continues with offering the vital organs of the pig to the ancestors: its heart, liver, and lungs. First, boys lay a second fire under the lower platform. A lot of dry twigs stir up the fire and cause heavy smoke. A curtain of fog lingers over the food garden. One of the boys puts a stick in the fire. One end is split in two and forms a Y-shape. Pieces of the pig's heart are stuck on both ends. Two other sticks are placed in the fire, one with a piece of liver and the other with part of the lungs. The organs are left in the fire to roast, and will be offered to the ancestors later in the ceremony.

Young men are still busy cutting the meat, and Maria stuffs the bamboo canes. Those which are ready are put in the fire to be cooked. More leaves cover the sago bundles, which steam in the smoke of the underlying fire. Children run around gnawing on a pig's foot, or play with its eyes, stuck on sticks. Adults sit together, engaged in lively conversation, waiting patiently for the food to be done.

Some twenty minutes later, Maria and Matius get up, take two larger bamboo stalks and walk a little way into the food garden, up to there where the vegetation begins. Firmly, they put the canes in the ground, crosswise. Agus joins

Maria and Matius. In one hand he holds three bundles of sago. In the other he holds the sticks with pieces of the heart, liver, and lungs. The three relatives stand close together, Agus in the middle, with their backs turned to the others. Then Agus calls his ancestors, one by one, loud and clear. By doing this, he invites each of them to come and eat the food they have prepared. When Agus is done, he puts the stuffed leaves and the spits with organs on the intersecting stalks. Maria and Matius put the bundles with sago they hold on the ground, so that they lean against the bamboo cross. For a moment Agus, Maria, and Matius stand there silent, deep in thought, before they turn back to the others.

This is the sign for the men and children to open the smoked, stuffed leaves that are left on the platform. The fire beneath is extinguished. Arit and two young men chop open the blackened roasted bamboo canes, take out the meat mixed with vegetables, and put it on the open folded sago leaves. All that time, Agus sits once more at the top of the ladder, on the small porch of the garden house, overlooking his relatives and the food garden.

Matius takes a leaf of one of the sago bundles, tears off a piece, and puts a portion of steaming pork and some sago on it. He then calls the names of the persons present, and they step forward. One by one, Matius hands everyone a portion of the cooked food, served on a leaf. Agus is the first to receive his share. Maria is next. After Arit follow all the other relatives, children included. Everybody looks for a place to sit down. Some sit on the ladder or join Agus on the small porch. Others take a seat on the muddy ground or climb up the platform.

Nobody finishes the served food. Symbolically they take one or two bites, then wrap it up in the leaves and tie the package with a liana. Suddenly, there is a lot of commotion. People walk up and down, starting to clear out the place. Matius and Maria take some opened bamboo tubes and bring them to the place where Agus offered the food for the ancestors. The remaining canes and sago bundles are divided among the people. Men check the smothered fires while women make sure the food garden is left nice and tidy. When people are ready, they take their carrierbags filled with food bundles and set off back to the village.

Agus, Maria, Matius and Arit are the last to go. Before they leave, they take a last look at the food garden. Silently they go on their way. Soon it will be sunset and darkness will settle on the village and its surroundings. The time has come for the ancestors to "come down."

When everyone has left the food garden and peace returns, the ancestors are given the opportunity to come and visit the place to eat the offered food. It is said that when the ancestors have eaten their share, and are pleased, they will return to their mountain in *seweron* and will stop interfering in the lives and health of their descendants. For safety's sake, so as not to disturb the peace and quiet and to give the ancestors free rein, the clan members will not work in their food garden for some weeks. The section behind the intersecting canes is, out of bounds until the food is consumed.

The next morning, Agus feels remarkably better. His fever abates and he has a good appetite. That week he gains some weight and feels much stronger. Agus stays with his sister and her family for four more weeks before he sets off for his home village. During that time he does not take any medicine whatsoever. When he is ready to depart, Agus is the same strong, healthy man he always has been. The nurses at the hospital are amazed when Agus comes to say good-bye. To them it seems like a miracle. But Agus knows better: the ancestors have returned home and so can he.

Agus has fulfilled his ceremonial obligations. He has given a festive meal to reassure the ancestors that the sacred cloth returned safely. By doing so, he has reconciled his spiritual and kinship relations, and in return is cured.

## CONCLUDING REMARKS

By exploring the performance of the Manes Kaya rite, it was shown that blood is the central humor in this healing rite. By examining the rite in terms of spiritual and kinship relations, it was further shown that blood, food, and sacred cloths are interconnected symbols.

The importance of food during the Manes Kaya ritual is expressed in various ways. In northwest Ayfat, food is used as a form of communication. People establish and confirm relationships, not only between relatives but especially with regard to the ancestors, by sharing and offering food. Further, food also refers to notions about sickness and health. People offer food in the context of rituals associated with sickness and misfortune. In northwest Ayfat, in case the illness is caused by ancestral spirits, being ill is seen as similar to being "eaten up." Therefore, people offer food, inviting the ancestors to come and eat the food instead. In accepting with thanks, the ancestors will, in return, restore one's health. The patient, then, can recover, which means that the condition of the blood regains its balance.

Blood not only is a central notion with regard to sickness and health, it also refers to social and kinship relations. The sick person defines who will attend the healing ritual and eat the offered food. Only blood relatives of the sick person can participate in the healing rite and consume the food. According to indigenous notions, the spirits of the ancestors would be upset if the food were served to nonrelatives. Consequently, the ancestors would withhold their assistance in curing the patient, or even punish the nonkin, who subsequently would be taken ill. The significance of blood relations also finds expression in the central role of sacred cloths, which are meant to stay within the lineage and are inherited from generation to generation.

To make sure no other people attend the healing rite, clan-bound healing rituals are generally performed in the food gardens, away from the village. Moreover, the food gardens are clan property, so the ground is connected with the ancestors. It is the correct way to worship the ancestors on their own territory, and to give and share food (that is sago, which is supposed to come from ancestral land) on clan ground.

Further, healing rituals are performed in the late afternoon. This is done not only because illness is associated with a "hot" state of the body, and the aim of the ritual is to "cool down" (that is to cure), the patient, but also because the spirits "come down" and visit the world of the living after sunset: this time not to haunt or frighten, a person, but to enjoy a festive dinner.

## NOTES

1. I conducted anthropological field research on female ritual healers in the northwest Ayfat region for thirteen months in 1994 and 1995, as a research associate of the Centre for Pacific Studies, Department of Anthropology, University of Nijmegen, and of ISIR, the NWO (Netherlands Organization for Scientific Research) priority program "The Irian Jaya Studies: A Program for Interdisciplinary Research," an interuniversity research project (coordinated by Leiden University), financed by WOTRO (Netherlands Foundation for the Advancement of Tropical Research). Financial support has been granted by ISIR and the Department of Anthropology, University of Nijmegen. The research was carried out in close cooperation with my friend and colleague anthropologist Louise Thoonen, who conducted research on female initiation and Christianity. I would like to thank Louise for her thorough and stimulating comments on earlier drafts of this chapter.

2. The Catholic mission entered the Ayfat area in 1949. Ayawasi became its center in the Ayfat region. Nowadays, Indonesian sisters are stationed in Ayawasi. For further reading on the arrival of the Catholic mission, see Thoonen 1998.

3. Manes Kaya literally means: "to bundle for the spirits of the deceased ancestors." The ritual is also called Aufenes, which means "bundle sago."

4. Every lineage posseses a number of cloths (***kain timur***). There are two kinds: sacred cloths (***kain pusaka***), which are inherited from generation to generation and are meant to stay within the clan, and cloths (***kain jalan***) used for (ceremonial) exchange within and between lineages. For further reading on ***kain timur***, see Elmberg 1968; Schoorl 1979; Miedema 1984; Haenen 1991.

5. I agree with Buckley and Gottlieb (1988), who argue that most anthropological studies on blood have been limited by exploring (menstrual) blood in terms of "taboo" and symbolic "pollution."

6. Ancestral spirits can wander to other, more faraway places. They remain, for instance, at holy places such as sacred mountains.

7. Although it is common to use *bofiet* as an herbal remedy, an overdose can easily kill a person. It was generally used by initiated men to take revenge on their enemies.

8. In the northwest Ayfat area, women hold the cloths under trust.

9. The ***kain timur*** Agus is talking about is ***wan Fas***. This cloth belongs to the category ***kain pusaka***.

10. The following ancestors are called upon: Kait, Wian, Sekiah, Nsudmbawew, Pofitsteyuo, Faw, Faye, Siendepo, Matiaf, Syewon, Haenebuoh, Sun Wakus.

11. The spirits of the ancestors of the Baru clan are believed to stay on the sacred mountain Faumair.

## REFERENCES

Baddeley, J. 1985. Traditional healing practices of Rarotonga, Cook Islands. In C. Parsons, ed., *Healing Practices in the South Pacific*, pp. 129–143. Honolulu: University of Hawaii Press.

Buckley, T., and A. Gottlieb (eds.). 1988. *Blood Magic: The Anthropology of Menstruation.* Berkeley and Los Angeles: University of California Press.

Courtens, I. 1998. As one woman to the other: Female ritual healers in northwest Ayfat. In J. Miedema et al., eds., *Perspectives on the Bird's Head of Irian Jaya, Indonesia: Proceedings of the Conference, Leiden, 13–17 October 1997*, pp. 33–50. Amsterdam and Atlanta: Rodopi.

Elmberg, J. 1968. *Balance and Circulation: Aspects of Tradition and Change Among the Mejprat of Irian Barat.* Monograph Series, Publication no. 12. Stockholm: Statens Etnografiska Museet.

Haenen, P. 1991. *Weefsels van wederkerigheid: Sociale structuur bij de Moi van Irian Jaya.* Ph.D. thesis, University of Nijmegen.

Haiveta, C. 1990. Health Care Alternatives in Maindroin. In N. Lutkehaus, ed., *Sepik Heritage: Tradition and Change in Papua New Guinea*, pp. 439–446. Durham, NC: Carolina Academic Press.

Keck, V. 1992. *Falsch gehandelt, schwer erkrankt.* Institute of Ethnology University of Beiträge zur Ethnologie 35. Basel.

Laderman, C., and M. Roseman (eds.). 1996. *The Performance of Healing.* New York and London: Routledge.

Macpherson, C. 1985. Samoan Medicine. In C. Parsons, ed., *Healing Practices in the South Pacific*, pp. 1–15. Honolulu: University of Hawaii Press.

Mageo, J., and A. Howard (eds.). 1996. *Spirits in Culture, History and Mind.* New York & London: Routledge.

Miedema, J. 1984. *De Kebar 1855–1980: Sociale structuur en religie in de Vogelkop van West-Nieuw-Guinea.* Dordrecht, Netherlands: ICG Printing.

Mitchell, W. 1990. Therapeutic systems of the Taute Wape. In N. Lutkehaus ed., *Sepik Heritage: Tradition and Change in Papua New Guinea*, pp. 428–438. Durham, NC: Carolina Academic Press.

Parsons, C. (ed.) 1985. *Healing Practices in the South Pacific.* Honolulu: University of Hawaii Press.

Schieffelin, E. 1996. On failure and performance: Throwing the medium out of the seance. In C. Laderman and M. Roseman, eds., *The Performance of Healing*, pp. 59–89. New York and London: Routledge.

Schoorl, H. 1979. *Mensen van de Ayfat: Ceremoniële ruil en sociale orde in Irian Jaya, Indonesia.* Ph.D. dissertation, University of Nijmegen.

Stephen, M. (ed.) 1987. *Sorcerer and Witch in Melanesia.* New Brunswick, NJ: Rutgers University Press.

Strathern, A., and P. Stewart. 1999. *Curing and Healing: Medical Anthropology in Global Perspective.* Durham, NC: Carolina Academic Press.

Thoonen, L. 1998. We have accepted the father first: The arrival of the Catholic Church in northwest Ayfat. In J. Miedema et al., eds., *Perspectives on the Bird's Head of Irian Jaya, Indonesia: Proceedings of the Conference, Leiden, 13–17 October 1997*, pp. 51–79. Amsterdam and Atlanta: Rodopi.

Trompf, G. 1991. *Melanesian Religion.* Cambridge: Cambridge University Press.

# CHAPTER 4

# A Comparative Discussion of Witchcraft and Healing Rituals

*Pamela J. Stewart and Andrew Strathern*

In this chapter we explore the materials from the Bird's Head of Irian Jaya presented in Chapters 2 and 3, and compare and contrast our materials from the Pangia, Duna, and Hagen areas of Papua New Guinea. Clearly, many historical, ecological, and geographical differences exist between the Bird's Head and the Highlands of Papua New Guinea, but our aim is to look at the fundamental notions of humors and substances that exist in these New Guinea areas as a comparative exercise and also as a contribution to the understanding of phenomenologically shaped concepts of the body/mind complex.

The Inanwatan and Ayfat case studies, in Chapters 2 and 3, cast interesting comparative shadows eastward to Papua New Guinea. In thematic terms, they contain between them a whole string of topics relating to the body, morality, the cosmos, humors and substances, emanations, food, sorcery and witchcraft, sickness, sacrifice, and the ancestors. Most importantly, they show how all of those topics are related and are mediated through aspects and conditions of the human body in its corelation and coexistence with others.

Seeing the body in this way implies that we see it both relationally and individually, as we have pointed out previously (Strathern and Stewart 1999). The whole emphasis on humors and substances indicates that the person's internal and external relations are symbolized in this way. The body has its boundaries in the skin, yet the skin is also the permeable integument through which substances and influences pass in both directions. Van Oosterhout (Chapter 2) makes particularly good use of this point in pursuing the questions of how

Inanwatan witches are said to operate and of how healings from witchcraft are attempted. It is in the conjunction of sweat and smell that the distinguishing features of the Inanwatan ideas emerge, and both sweat and smell emerge from the internal body through the skin, thus becoming signs of inner states that are communicated to the outside world. The Duna of Papua New Guinea say that the inner state of witches is revealed by the fact that they are unable to cry or have difficulty in producing tears at funerals. This is a particularly troubling inability because Duna women form mourning groups that attend funerals, where they are expected to express the grief of the community at large. Sometimes these groups can be heard wailing as they move along pathways leading from their parish to that of the funeral. Those who are seen to be standing outside of this custom might be subject to witchcraft accusations. The singing of these laments is accompanied by crying, which is thought to encourage the spirit (*tini*) of the dead person to journey to its appropriate dwelling place high in the forested areas above the villages. Two examples of these songs follow:

> My child, will you come back
> Like the *yope* bird, sometime?
> Will you come like a *yope* bird
> To the place Laki?
> My son, like a parakeet
> For which a trap has been placed,
> Do not think back,
> My son, like a parakeet
> For which a trap has been placed,
> Go to Yapi and Yapale,
> Do not think back.
> My daughter, like a ribbon-tail bird,
> Wearing your little apron,
> Go to Angana and Angakana.
> My daughter, like a sicklebill bird,
> Go up to Yapi and Yawepi, up there,
> Where the rock stands out. (Stewart and Strathern 2000)

Here the mother had recently lost a small son and daughter in an epidemic of sickness following a severe drought in the Aluni Valley in 1998. She compares both children to birds and tells them to fly up to mountain cave sites, the abodes of the dead (Laki, Yapi, Yapale, etc.), and stay there. She sang the lament at the funeral of an old man who had passed away. Women sing these songs at grave sites as well as at funeral gatherings, where the women huddle around the body of the deceased, wailing and singing lament songs. Each woman sings to the souls of her own dead kinfolk, telling them to greet the new arrival and assist in making the *tini* of the recently dead person feel welcome and at home in the community of the dead. (This custom of sending one's tears with a newly dead person's soul back to the spirits of kinfolk who have died is known also in the Hagen and Pangia areas.) The dead all belong together in the same place, and the recent dead must continually be sent back to their new, wild forest dwelling places in the limestone cliffs high above the dwellings of the living.

In another lament on the same occasion, the woman U. sang as follows:

> Where shall I go?
> My father, shall I be like an *umi* bird,
> A child of the places Kwane and Kewane?
>
> My father, I, your last-born child,
> At the places Poko and Payako,
> With whom shall I go to live?
>
> My father, at the places Poko and Payako,
> I, your last-born, see
> You are not there anymore.
>
> . . .
>
> My father, did you make
> A little house at Apanda,
> At Kira, at Kirapi,
> To sleep there like a cassowary?
>
> My father, at the places Yawe and Yapale,
> When the *alo* bird calls out crossly,
> Will you return in the afternoon?
>
> My father, you must go
> To your mother's place, where
> The red-plumed bird of paradise calls,
> You must go and stay.
>
> My father, take hold of your stick,
> Walk slowly up
> To the places Laki and Lakiya. (Stewart and Strathern 2000)

The woman here mourns for her newly dead father and refers to the fact that she is married and lives in her husband's parish, apart from the father. She names the small places where she lives, Kwane and Kewane, Poko and Payako, grouping them in pairs. Such a form of naming is often used honorifically in songs, dignifying a single place by giving it two names and so giving it a cadence of plurality. Later she sings of Kira and Kirapi, Yawe and Yapale, Laki and Lakiya, all secondary burial places in the parish territory of her dead father, to which he belonged through his mother. The constant reference to bird calls indicates the sense of community between birds of the forest and people, reflecting also the idea that the souls of the dead can take the form of birds and communicate with people.

Returning to the discussion of smell, van Oosterhout makes a further point: that people are in a sense unambiguously defined by smell. The Inanwatan say that they share food from the same ancestral ground, and therefore they have the same flesh and the same scent or smell. As long as they stay on their ground, then, and eat the same foods from it, their flesh and smell will (by implication) stay the same. By the same token, this identity is potentially mutable, because if they moved elsewhere and/or ate other foods, it would change. Nothing could indicate more sharply the coexistence of ideas of permanence with ideas of mutability that is found widely in New Guinea in contexts of identity formation.

Thus, we see that ideas of identity through food are not sharply opposed to those of identity through blood or descent, because these are interrelated in an overall cycle, what for Hagen in Papua New Guinea has been called the grease cycle (Strathern 1974, 1982), and for which we can read the fertility cycle (see Chapter 5 for further elaboration on this point). We see the Hagen grease or *kopong* as being equivalent in many aspects to the concept in Inanwatan of *iware*, which van Oosterhout refers to as life force, encompassing power, sacral knowledge, and creativity as well as physical procreation. Such a set of ideas tells us again that we are dealing with holistic notions that function as overarching principles of social life and visions of the cosmos at the same time. We can say, then, that the human body is relational not just in the sense of being a site for the expression or impression of social relationships. It is also a part of a much wider life world in which the world as a whole is constantly in processes of decay and renewal. The "fractal" or "self-similar" features of a world conceived of in these terms (Wagner 1991; Gell 1998) derive their dynamic, therefore, not simply from ideas of logical similarity but also from the flows of substance that actually link people to their world, so that aspects of the body pass into the world and vice versa, in a mutually sustaining and defining fashion.

In Inanwatan, ancestral essence is in the ground and permeates food, which then builds flesh and blood. In turn, the moral state of the person impacts on the body, causing it to exude sweat and smell. These then become markers of that moral state. Alternatively, sorcerers and witches, representing destructive, aggressive, and consuming forces, can alter the body's internal state and therefore cause it to sweat differently or smell different. The Inanwatan *suangi* (witch) places rotting leaves inside a victim, and the smell of these announces the fact.

Interestingly, this detail dovetails with observations regarding assault sorcery in many cases from elsewhere in New Guinea. For example, the *uro* sorcerers in Pangia in Papua New Guinea stuff leaves into the abdomen of the victim, having first removed vital organs, and then place a kidney in the mouth of the victim (Stewart and Strathern 1997, 1999b). The dazed victim takes the kidney home, roasts it in the fire, and eats it, committing autocannibalism:

confusing inside with outside, consuming personal substance rather than nurturing it, in a forced self-victimization. The witch among the Duna of Papua New Guinea is thought to consume the inner organs as well as to stuff the body with leaves. In Hagen rumors have arisen from time to time that witchcraft is being spread like an infection, in one instance through the placing of human flesh in streams and the consumption of its "grease" by people who drink the water from these sources (Stewart and Strathern 1999b). Among the Duna, the fear that witches are multiplying is linked to latter-day notions that witches are the instruments of Satan, whose powers are growing in the "end times" before the millennium (Stewart and Strathern 1999a, 1999d).

In both cases the secrecy/revelation scenario that is basic to witchcraft is conducive to suspicion of a covert increase in danger. The Duna have revived the use of their traditional divining stick (*ndele rowa*) in an attempt to identify and control witches. Interestingly, the stick is festooned with nut shells from the *Pangium edule* tree. The shells rattle as the stick is carried, advertising where it is being carried to; but they are also a reminder of the highly prized and strong-smelling fruit itself, analogous to the "meat" that witches are said to crave. The Duna, in fact, have their own way of either appeasing a discovered witch or "curing" her. The witch can be offered pork and asked to desist from eating the human flesh of the victim; or the witch may confess to an act of witchcraft and thereafter is supposed not to commit such an act again. In the past, confession also usually enabled the witch to avoid being put to death. Thus, the career of a given witch can be ended. The tendency to witchcraft is replicated, however, by its reappearance over the generations, carried in the bodies of those descended from witches and hidden there until it reveals itself in adulthood (Strathern and Stewart 1999; Stewart and Strathern 1999b). The ordered cosmos thus contains the seeds of disorder and of conflict.

A narrative given in the 1990s by a knowledgeable senior Duna man, A., clearly exemplifies several of these points. His story tells of a ritual expert who was imbued with the power to divine for witches and was able to use the *ndele rowa*, which would smell the odor of a witch and could identify her by striking the ground and vibrating so that the attached nut shells loudly sounded out the discovery.

### The Ritual Expert Who Could Divine for Witches

This man went to the mountainous areas and ate the *arikombo* fruit—a good-smelling fruit. He climbed up the tree and sang loudly, calling out the names of all the mountains and creeks in the area. He held on to the tree with one arm and with the other shook it violently. He asked that the female spirits who lived in the places that he called the names of should come and make him strong by coming inside of him. After this he returned to his house, and at night he heard the female creatures [*aruatome*] that he had called. Then he was able to use the *ndele rowa* to divine for witches. . . . If a witch had killed someone, then the *ndele rowa* would hit the ground and follow the footsteps of the witch. The prints might appear as those of a cassowary or a wild pig, but these were actually the witch's.

The witch would have wanted to kill a person, and in doing so would have buried a stick called a *pepe rowa* in a hidden area. The *ndele rowa* would move along until it had discovered the place where this marker of the witch's intention was. When the ritual expert was led to this place by the *ndele rowa*, he would see a small sign, such as a broken area of ground, and he would say, "Dig here, and you will find the *pepe rowa.*" Then the *ndele rowa* would lead the expert to the house of the witch. The path leading to this woman's house would then be marked by the expert with a stick. He would not confront the woman immediately. He would go and find the parents and husband and other family members of the woman and tell them to go and get this woman. He would go along back to her house, and the *ndele rowa* would indicate which woman in the house was the witch. The *ndele rowa* could smell the witch. All those present would ask the woman why she had killed a person who was not a tribal enemy. Men would gather around and encircle her and ask her why she did this act. Eventually, she would say that she had desired to do it.

At the time of her confession, men with short tempers might kill the witch by shooting her with an arrow, or they might allow her to have another chance at life if she agreed not to kill again. If she was allowed to live, a big pig would be killed and the neck bone [a prized piece of pork] would be given to her to eat, and she would be told to eat pork meat and not human meat. Then the men would show her two arrows and say, "If you kill again, we will use these arrows to kill you, or if we do not shoot you then you will be given a cane rope and you can hang yourself [suicide by hanging is not uncommon in the Duna area]. If you don't want to kill yourself with cane rope, then we will provide you with a pig's rope. If you do not want to die, then do not kill again." Thus a woman might be given a chance to live even after confessing to using witchcraft to kill someone. When a woman did kill herself by hanging, an examination of her body would be made to see if her heart was enlarged and filled with black blood—a sign that she had killed and eaten humans. [If the woman's heart was not seen to be enlarged or particularly black, then it would be said that she was actually not a witch and compensation would subsequently have to be given to her family.]

Here we see the theme of odor as a marker of social behavior and its ensuing bodily condition, as discussed also by van Oosterhout for the Inanwatan people (see Chapter 2).

The witches in Duna are said to "eat" their victims as an expression of inappropriate and unconstrained desire for meat. In the above narrative, pork meat was offered to the witch so that she would be satisfied and might modify her behavior so as to conform to socially accepted consumption modes. The story of witches eating human meat instead of nonhuman animal meat finds its parallel in narratives of early mythological times, when some humans supposedly routinely ate human meat and were unfamiliar with the practice of eating pork until they were taught to put salt on pork meat and to bury the bodies of dead humans.

Steadman (1971) describes a similar situation in his ethnography of the Hewa people (the northern neighbors of the Duna), where "death attributed to a killing by a witch, *pisai mai* (witch eaten), is considered a subcategory of *miniam* [death caused by sickness or old age]" (p. 203). During the 1960s witchcraft accusations were often made against the women in the Hewa community where Steadman was working, but these did not generally lead to the woman being killed. If the woman was killed, a *postmortem* would be conducted, as was done in the Duna area, to look for signs to indicate whether the woman was actually a witch or not (p. 209). Sometimes men were accused of being witches (p. 244), as is also true in the Duna area. Hewa witches are said to harbor inappropriate desires to consume human flesh, which leads to their actions.

Appropriate and inappropriate consumption are important themes throughout New Guinea. Eating is the locus of nurture and kinship. Yet a sorcerer can poison a victim with a gift of food; and a witch eats the victim instead of giving nurture. In turn, witches are universally said to attack victims because of jealousy over a failure to share food. Such ideas strengthen and weaken social relations at the same time, and they relate to the same overall conceptions of the flow and consolidation or surcease and depletion of fertility in the broadest sense.

This point, that ideas of witchcraft and sorcery relate to the same basic worldview as ideas regarding tutelary spirits and ancestors, and these in turn to notions of the flow of life force in the cosmos, can be supported by comparing van Oosterhout's discussion of sickness caused by *suangi* witchcraft and Courtens's account of a healing ceremony carried out to appease the ancestors in west Ayfat (Chapter 3). In the west Ayfat case the ancestors had not been informed about a cloth transaction that had taken place within the group, and they had to be placated by being shown the cloths and given a sacrifice of pork and other food. They were said to have caused the sickness by "eating" the insides of the sick man. In Inanwatan, during *suangi* sickness a witch may eat a vital part of the victim that is expressive of identity. But the *suangi* witch is seen as a living outsider, whereas the Ayfat ancestor is a deceased insider. The idiom of sickness causation is the same, but the social context is different. The witch acts unreciprocally, "steals," whereas the ancestor putatively enforces reciprocity and receives a "sacrifice," a gift. It is interesting that both Inanwatan witch and Ayfat ancestor are said to "eat" people and cause them to fall ill, and the sacrifice offered to the ancestors is in a sense given instead of the vitality of the sick person. This is exactly what was done to appease Duna witches in the past. We suggest that the distinction between ancestor and witch corresponds to the contrast Edmund Leach (1961) drew between "controlled supernatural attack" and "uncontrolled mystical influence," whereas the parallel between them rests on the image of "eating" in a world defined by the need for reciprocity and balance in a field of life force.

The image of eating applied to both witchcraft and ancestral attack is widespread in New Guinea. For example, in Pangia the ghosts of kin were said to "strike and eat" (*wia nako*) persons, making them sick, in order to induce them to make sacrifices. In general, the boundary between ancestors and witches may become blurred: ancestors, too, may be arbitrary and malevolent, difficult to please. There is an "outside" aspect to them, because they are dead, and an "inside" one, because they are kin. Witches are usually seen as "outside" attackers, yet they are also in a sense "inside," for example, when those accused of witchcraft are likely to be women in-married into a local group, as happens with the Inanwatan of Irian Jaya and the Duna of Papua New Guinea.

Such a combination of inside and outside characteristics provides the vehicle for the idea that witches may make hidden attacks on the unseen inner parts of a victim, just as ancestral ghosts do. And the "site" where evidence of such an attack shows is on the skin, the locus of external moral information. The skin is where that which is invisible is made visible. Van Oosterhout points out, for example, that acts of stealing cause people to have bad skin. In the same way people in Pangia say that long hairs growing on the skin of a person's pigs are an indication that the person has done some hidden wrong. The hairs are a sign that the pig's vitality is diverted into the hairs rather than into making consumable flesh; the hairs are singed off when the pig is cooked. Long hairs also make the pig like a wild, rather than a domesticated, creature. The pig is here equated with, or stands for, its owner, reflecting in itself the condition of the owner, externalizing the owner's hidden internal condition. In Hagen the skin is thought to reflect the inner emotional state of a person, and feelings such as shame or anger are said to show themselves on the skin (Strathern 1975; Strathern and Stewart 1999).

This view of the skin should not lead us to accept a purely textualist version of the body. Van Oosterhout's account is replete with references to physiological facts and processes—including sweat, smell, body weight, putrefaction, health and sickness—that both ground the body in experience (see Csordas 1994) and at the same time carry import for symbolic schemes of value. The social body is at one and the same time the physical body, and its physiological processes constantly feed into the symbolic interpretations of it. Without sweat and smell, the Inanwatan symbolic universe would be greatly altered. Similarly, in Pangia, anger is described as ***korimi***, a "stink" (corresponding to the English-language metaphor). Stink also attaches to that which is rotten: meat that has gone bad and has a putrid smell, also described as ***korimi***. ***Korimi*** as anger is said to be located in the nose, which of course is also the organ of smell. For the Pangia people, then, "bad smell" is both a part of their sensate world and a part of their symbolic universe, closely paralleling Inanwatan ideas. They, too, recognize that the sensate, nonverbal world provides a check on verbal statements and that people practice verbal trickery to conceal their true feelings but other forms of evidence reveal these.

As noted earlier, van Oosterhout provides us with information about skin changing that belongs to this part of the discussion (see also Strathern 1996; Tuzin 1997). She points out that the theme of hiding the real skin and of skin changing belongs to the sense of trickery in life. Confusion of identity may arise when one modality of information negates another or when there is an inappropriate mixing of substances. It may also arise as a result of purposeful action. Van Oosterhout tells us that the Inanwatan nowadays extend this idea to God, whom they describe as appearing to be an old man with a dry, ugly, and smelly skin who begs for food. Those with insight can see through this disguise to his true nature. New Guinea mythologies are full of this theme of disguise which reinforces the notion that things may not be what they seem, and although the skin is supposed to reveal the person's nature, it may in fact be a camouflage. An example of the "removable skin" motif from the Hagen balladic genre known as *kang rom* is given here:

### The Story of Miti Krai and Ambra Amb Rangmba

Miti Krai sees a column of smoke in the distance at the Ambra sweet potato garden. He wants to investigate. His mother warns him of the potential dangers ahead for him traveling to unknown regions. But he goes off and at Ambra meets Rangmba and he and she declare that they will always be together as husband and wife. Just as Miti Krai and Rangmba are preparing to leave Ambra to return to Miti Krai's village where they will live, Rangmba transforms herself into an old, ugly female; but Miti Krai had promised always to be loyal to Rangmba, so he takes her on the long journey back home. Upon arrival at his home village his people are revolted by the old woman who is his wife since she is supposed to be a young bride able to work for many years and raise children. Miti Krai is scolded for bringing her home with him and his sister complains loudly and beats Rangmba severely. But Miti Krai takes Rangmba to his house and begins married life with her. One day a big man dies and a funeral is prepared for him. Before attending the funeral Rangmba transforms herself again, this time into a handsome young man. At the funeral Miti Krai's sister, the one who had beaten Rangmba when she first came home with Miti Krai, sees the handsome youth who is really Rangmba in a transformed state and she falls in love with the youth. Meanwhile, Miti Krai goes ahead and prepares a large bridewealth payment, having seen a speck of red ochre paint on Rangmba's eyelid as a mark of her former appearance. Rangmba eludes Miti Krai's sister and in secret transforms herself back into a young beautiful female—the one that Miti Krai had first seen and fallen in love with. The sister of Miti Krai who had treated Rangmba so badly was heart broken and unable to recover herself. (Strathern and Stewart 1997:6)

The narrative clearly indicates the theme that surface appearances may be deceptive, and that by responding only to these and not considering things more carefully, people may make mistakes. But the story's structure also tells us about the close relationship between opposite-sex siblings and the potential opposition between sisters-in-law. It also suggests the interchangeability of the generations (old and young) and the sexes (female and male). The one emerges out of the other and may merge back; but at the end of the narrative the desired final transformation of identity occurs when Rangmba once more becomes the vital young woman whom Miti Krai had courted so ardently.

Another example of the "removable skin" motif from the Duna area tells of a *tama* (spirit) that lived at a place called Bakalikako at Yeru in the Strickland River valley:

### The Story of the Flying Fox

On a night when a man went hunting for a flying fox [a fruit bat], a young woman appeared as he waited. He took the hand of the woman and they went to his house. She married the man, and together they had ten children. One day the husband went to the south, toward the Huli area, in order to obtain salt. Upon leaving he instructed his family to watch the *hale suko* banana tree, telling them that if the fruit of the tree pointed to their house, he would be safe, but if the tree itself leaned in a different direction, he would be in danger somewhere.

The family watched the tree, and it pointed toward the house and the bananas on it became ripe. Time passed, and one of the man's sons picked bananas from the tree and ate them. The other sons followed the example of the first son and began eating bananas from the tree, so that by the time the father returned home, there were no bananas left at all. . . . When he saw that all the bananas on the tree were gone, he turned to his wife and exclaimed, "You are not a real woman—you can turn into other things. You turned into a flying fox, as did your children, and you ate my bananas." The husband stormed off to rest after his long journey and subsequent outburst of anger.

While he slept, the wife took all their children and left. After traveling a long way, she and the children reached a large limestone sinkhole which was so deep that when sticks were thrown into it, the sound of them hitting the bottom was not heard. The mother took a stick and broke the shoulders of each of her sons and threw them, one after the other, into the hole, where they turned into flying foxes. Then she broke her own shoulders and jumped into the hole, where she transformed back into a flying fox. The husband was grieved at what had happened, and cried and cried until at last he turned into a cockatoo bird the cry of which is *hale, hale, hale* [the name of the banana tree in the story]. (K.; May 1991).

Here the young woman the man meets is a transformed version of a flying fox or fruit bat. These bats are fond of bananas, and by implication the woman's sons who eat the bananas, contrary to the father's command, show their batlike maternal nature in this uncontrolled consumption. When the husband directly accuses his wife of showing her "true" nature, she takes him at his word and transforms her children and herself into actual bats. The narrative does not directly speak of a removable skin but of a bodily transformation. The wife is a spirit wife, able to shift her shape from bat to woman and back again. Moral behavior is at stake and is tested, as in the Hagen story. Those who fail the test are left unhappy. Accusing someone of not being what they purport to be can itself be morally unacceptable and bring retribution. The latent moral, like that of the class of stories to which this one belongs, is that husbands need to treat their wives and children with respect and care, and not regard them as outsiders or "wild things." If they do not, they may elicit or provoke the return of an actual "wild" identity. The prototype in all the stories about the shape-changing wife is the powerful female spirit, the Payame Ima, who protects both sexes against the hidden powers of witchcraft (see Stewart and Strathern 1999c).

The "removable skin" motif represents the transformable aspects of the person, indicating that a person may be handsome beneath and ugly on the surface, or vice versa. Here we see how the senses can be fooled. A "false" visual image can be seen that at the metaphysical level represents the state of flow which humans, animals, and elements of the environment are continually in. This imagery of the transformer figure is very common in New Guinea (see Strathern and

Stewart 2000b; Tuzin 1997) and is emblematic of a fundamental principle of continuity of humankind with other life forms and the cosmos at large.

This motif may further be tied to the widespread idea in Irian Jaya of the snake-man, who can change his skin as snakes do but is a handsome man beneath the disguise of his snake skin. (The idea also appears among the Duna.) This snake may be the source of all renewal and restoration of fertility, as in the myth of Ambonai from Biak in Irian Jaya (Kamma 1972:70–71). Casting the Christian God in the role of the camouflaged deity who tests his potential followers and rewards those who can recognize his true nature therefore is clearly a mythological move that links Christian ideas to indigenous notions of reversal and renewal mediated by alterations in skin (compare Robbins 1997). The power of reversals is also pointed to by van Oosterhout (Chapter 2) when she writes of the ritual preparations that were thought necessary to survive an impending great flood: the Inanwatan were to hide inside their houses, isolating themselves and hoarding food supplies, in a reversal of normal behavior that would prevent the flood from capturing them. In a parallel to this notion, the Duna and Huli peoples thought that at the time of a cataclysmic ash fall they must gather inside a special house, reverse the ordinary ways of living, and thus survive, bringing normality back through the careful observance of taboos. In liminal times, such reversals of behavior are seen as ways of surviving challenges and also of switching the cosmos into a new pattern.

Predictably, food taboos are prominently observed at such liminal times. In Hagen such taboos marked out the bodies of cult participants as being in a special ritual state (Stewart and Strathern 1999c). If we recall that the emphasis on food and nurture as a source of identity is widespread in New Guinea, as elsewhere, then it is clear that observing rules of abstinence by definition sets one apart from others by inducing a change in one's body, thereby also fitting it for the ritual activity. Both the Inanwatan and the Ayfat show this pattern (Chapters 2 and 3). Food may be transformed into blood or blood and grease or water/vital essence throughout New Guinea (compare the Hua concept of *nu*; Meigs 1984). And these substances, we may say, correspond to the reproductive fluids or humors that define the creation of new human beings via sexual intercourse. Through this nexus of ideas, we wish to stress, it is again apparent that identity through descent and identity through locality merge. Food and its transformations mediate these two principles, making them one.

Such ideas are likely to persist in New Guinea societies, albeit with alterations in emphasis, through circumstances of historical change such as the coming of Christianity. Indeed, these circumstances may be described in terms of older concepts of the cosmos, as when the Duna (like the Inanwatan) perceive an increase in the prevalence of witchcraft and describe this as a result of the loss of secret knowledge and the weakening of rules that regulate sexual relations. The work of indigenous healers may be suspended because of Christianity, but can also reappear in a "camouflaged" form reminiscent of the general theme of camouflaging and renewal mentioned above. Thus, among the Duna witch finders have reappeared under the guise or label of "prophets." In the past they were imbued with their specific divinatory powers by female spirits; now it is said that God gives this power to chosen men. In Hagen, pastors of the charismatic churches take on healing roles, replacing the indigenous healers, all of whom converted to Christianity and interpreted this as meaning that they should no longer practice their trade or transmit their knowledge to successors. "Anita," a Hagen woman who was working as a ritual expert in the 1960s and whom we interviewed in 1998, declared that when she became a Catholic, she decided to stop her ritual work, though she was very proud of her memories of it and of the material goods and prestige her knowledge had brought her. This section can be compared with material presented by Ien Courtens in chapter 3 and the description of three ritual healers from the Mararoko Kewa area in Papua New Guinea described by MacDonald (1991:142–157).

## RITUAL EXPERTS AND BODY SUBSTANCES

Experts in ritual curing practices in Highlands societies of New Guinea dealt intimately with the flows and balances of substances in the body, either by directly manipulative actions or symbolically, in the words of their magical spells for curing. In the Duna area, healing powers were thought to be given to selected men and women through a close relationship with the category of female spirits known as Payame Ima. The knowledge of how to use various types of earth poultices along with incantations would be shared with a man or a woman after the female spirit had chosen the person and after he or she had proven to be loyal to her. If the relationship between the human and the spirit ended, the power to heal would be withdrawn from the healing expert.

In the Hagen area healing practitioners also could be either male or female. In 1998 we interviewed a woman who had been an expert in curing until she took up Christianity (Catholicism) some years ago. She had been active in her art in the clan territory of her husband near Mbukl and Golke in the 1960s and 1970s. We will call her Anita.

Anita is a strong character and proud of the work she had done as a curer. We asked how she had obtained her knowledge. "I myself found it" (*na nanom-nt kandep tit*), she replied. But the deeper background was that the knowledge came to her through the spirit of her dead father, who had been a "big man" or leader in his clan. The spirit returned to her in a dream, and told her that he was giving her this power of his, which he himself had practiced while he was alive. The knowledge came into her heart (*muntmong*) and went up into her chest, into her *noman* (mind). At this time she was a grown woman, married and the mother of a son. While her father was alive, he had mentioned his magical powers to her and had told her that later she would have two sons when she married. (She did indeed have two sons.) The father had four sons, all of whom grew up to be prominent men who made *moka* exchanges (see A. Strathern 1971 for an exposition of *moka*; and Strathern and Stewart 2000a for a historical discussion of changes in it over time.) She was his only daughter, and he liked her, she said, and so she "got his *noman*." She was the only one to get his ritual powers because of his liking for her. (The implication was that this was an act of personal favor from her father.) She eventually gave up her practice as a result of a later dream in which the Christian God commanded her to desist from it.

Anita specialized in the removal of intrusive and dangerous substances from the bodies of her patients. For example, she could remove sorcery substance from people's stomachs by rubbing them with special leaves and extracting the substance, tipping it into a bamboo tube. After this it was spread out and examined by kinfolk of the patient in order to guess where the patient had ingested it (and therefore who was responsible for administering it). The kinfolk called her in when the patient was at the point of death, but as soon as she removed the "poison stuff" (*konga*), the sick person recovered. For a service like this she was paid a large pig and a valuable pearl shell.

We asked Anita if she used spells. She said yes, but it was many years ago and she could not remember the precise details. (Because we were talking to her in her house, within earshot of her neighbors, she may have been embarrassed to recite the spells or may have been concerned to protect her original trade secrets.) She could recall elements of these spells. One was to call on the names of high mountains, such as Mt. Wilhelm in the Chimbu area to the east and Mt. Ialibu to the south. The "poison" was to be sent to these high, wild, remote areas. She also called on eels, red parrots, and the eagle. Eels are slippery, and the poison would slip out of the patient. Eagles drive things away from the places they occupy, and red parrots expel intruders to their nests, which are made in holes in trees. Thus all these things were used as images of expulsion and extrusion. Anita's list here closely parallels the kinds of symbolism found in the repertoires of other ritual experts. She did not make the patient vomit the stomach contents, but said she squeezed or gathered these through the surface of the skin, a skill only ritual experts possess. The idea of the body involved here is that just as hostile magic can inject things through body tissues, so curing magic, aided by the power of words in the spell coming from the curer's *noman*, can extract them. The body responds to the expert's physical touch.

The "poison" involved here could include the menstrual blood of a woman inadvertently or inappropriately ingested by a male patient either in food or in sexual intercourse. (Some informants in previous years had declared that Anita used to operate directly with her mouth on men's sexual organs to pull the blood out. Such a practice was not a part of her own narrative to us.)

Anita also performed one special service for women. This was magic to secure the sexual preference and attention of a husband and to drive away other women or wives: the magic of *wölik*, female competition. She gave special plants to women who consulted her with this need in mind. Two were herbs that she called *muripa* and *röu*. A woman took these and cooked them in food to be given to her husband so that, in case the man had another wife or other wives, he would prefer the one who had fed him this bespelled food. Whereas the treatment for "poison" was to remove it from the stomach, here the aim was to insert magical herbs into the stomach, which (like "poison") would lodge there and hold the husband's affections. The same basic idea is involved: that powers of life and death over people are contained in the act of giving food. The same term (*kopna* or *konga*, literally "ginger") is used to describe either lethal magic or magic to secure a person's affections and desires.

Anita explained that before removing sorcery substance from a patient, she spoke her magical spell into her hand, thus empowering this part of her body to remove the substance by rubbing and squeezing the patient's skin. The spell effectively transmitted what was in her *noman* (mind, will, intention), the permanent seat of her power. The *noman* originally "translated" (understood) the power that had come up in her heart as a result of the dream she was given by her dead father, and then it held the knowledge there. The force of her magic is thus seen as an extension of her personal knowledge and willpower, as well as being a gift from the dead parent.

From Anita's account it is clear that plants and leaves were an important adjunct to her practice. In removing menstrual blood, for example, she cooked onions and gave them to the man to eat. She named other plants that she used to strengthen her hand when massaging a patient's stomach, including the herb *roepa* that grows under a hoop pine tree, and went on to describe a concoction of plants that she inserted as spicing into a kind of "sausage" (*rondoka*) that was prepared when a pork sacrifice (made to dead kin) accompanied her curing activities. This concoction included leaves of the *malt* tree, *roepa*, and ginger root. The same concoction could be used along with magic to secure the affections of a sexual partner. Anita stressed that the magic for the affections was directly aimed at the *noman* of the person who was its object. Once the *noman* was affected in this way, she claimed, the results were permanent. A young woman could attract a man to her in this way; a husband on whom the magic was made would get rid of any other wives he had; if a husband was about to divorce his wife but ate her magic food, he would retain her and stay faithfully with her. Anita's art here clearly drew its popularity from the charged competitive context of the polygynous "big man" form of society. Her own father, she commented, had eight wives, and was a "big man" who needed wives in order to succeed in exchange transactions that required the labor of these wives.

Anita stressed that she received large amounts of pay for her curing and other magical services. She used the wealth she received to initiate cycles of *moka* exchanges. She was a "big woman" (*amb nuim*), just as her father was a "big man." Anita's claim here is notable, given the general supposition that women did not make *moka* as agents in their own right in the past. Her account contradicts this picture, which is generally given by men, and suggests that an exceptional woman could break the pattern. As was also the case with "big men" who held ritual powers of healing, Anita's capacities as a curer directly strengthened her ability to enter into the *moka* system, seen as a result of her strong *noman*. It is apparent also that there is a strong symbiosis between *noman* and body. The two are intertwined. Powers of mind, or agency, affect the body, and conditions of the body affect the mind. Hence the combination of the spell (*mön*), a product of the *noman*, and the material substances (*tamb mel*) that went with it.

Anita's new religion, Catholicism, is also classified as a kind of *mön* in the Hagen language, reflecting its emphasis on rites, incantations, and prayers.

In terms of the theme of images of the body, Anita's account indicates the central importance of the stomach and of giving food. Sorcery substance is lethal "food" (*röng*), severing life; magic for affection is also food, cooked by a woman and given with intent to the man of her choice, joining his life to hers. Sorcery substance attacks the flesh of the body and must be physically removed in order to effect a cure. Affection magic attacks the mind of its recipient, via the stomach, and according to Anita, once it had secured its place in the *noman*, it cannot be reversed, becoming a kind of "healing" for which there was, in this sense, no "cure."

In Courtens's Ayfat study the sick man, Agus, visits his sister Maria Baru, who is a healer, although also a longtime member of the Catholic Church. She presides over a ceremony for him, directed by what she has seen in a dream coming from the ancestors. In her dream she saw sacred cloths and a pig, which she interpreted as being the ancestors' call for a sacrifice. This Ayfat example shows how easy it would be conceptually for such a practice to reemerge in Hagen, where dreams are important in all contexts, Christian or otherwise, and where sicknesses are still referred to as the work of the ghosts of dead kin, although these are partly conflated now with "the Devil" as *kor kit*, "bad spirits." Nowadays in Hagen, Christian rituals of fasting and prayer are designed to influence the amalgam of body and spirit/mind that the Christian religion envisages as the person. Christian ideas have also somewhat "fixed" the cosmos in an absolute opposition between good and evil, seen rather differently than the older pattern of alternating flows of fertility/increase and destruction/depletion. We will find more examples of subtle ways in which indigenous and Christian ideas blend, deflect, and mutually transform each other when we look in some detail at Hagen ideas about the *noman* (mind) in Chapter 7.

We have mentioned how ideas of conception and reproduction form a part of a total system of ideas about the cosmos, realized to a great extent in notions of humors and substances. We consider this theme further in Chapter 5.

## REFERENCES

Csordas, Thomas (ed.). 1994. *Embodiment and Experience: The Existential Ground of Culture and Self.* Cambridge: Cambridge University Press.

Gell, Alfred. 1998. *Art and Agency.* Oxford: Clarendon Press.

Kamma, Freerk C. 1972. *Koreri. A Messianic Movement in the Biak–Numfor Area.* The Hague: Martinus Nijhoff.

Leach, Edmund R. 1961. *Rethinking Anthropology.* London School of Economics, Monograph no. 22. London: Athlone Press.

MacDonald, Mary N. 1991. *Mararoko. A Study in Melanesian Religion.* American University Studies Series XI, Anthropology and Sociology vol. 45. New York: Peter Lang.

Meigs, Anna. 1984. *Food, Sex, and Pollution: A New Guinea Religion.* New Brunswick, NJ: Rutgers University Press.

Robbins, Joel. 1997. 666, or why is the millennium on the skin? Morality, the state and the epistemology of apocalypticism among the Urapmin of Papua New Guinea. In Pamela J. Stewart, and Andrew Strathern, eds. n.d. *Millennial Markers*, pp. 35–58. Townsville, Queensland: James Cook University, Centre for Pacific Studies.

Steadman, Lyle B. 1971. *Neighbours and Killers: Residence and Dominance among the Hewa of New Guinea.* Ph.D thesis, Australian National University.

Stewart, Pamela J., and Andrew Strathern. 1997. Sorcery and sickness: Spatial and temporal movements in Papua New Guinea and Australia. Discussion Papers Series, no. 1, pp. 1–27. Townsville, Queensland: James Cook University, Centre for Pacific Studies.

Stewart, Pamela J., and Andrew Strathern. 1999a. Engendering the millennium in Papua New Guinea. In Brenda Brasher and Lee Quinby, eds., *Engendering the Millennium*, special issue of *Journal of Millennial Studies* 2(1). Electronic journal, Center for Millennial Studies (http://www.mille.org).

Stewart, Pamela J. and Andrew Strathern 1999b. "Feasting on my enemy": Images of violence and change in the New Guinea highlands. *Ethnohistory* 46(4):645–669.

Stewart, Pamela J., and Andrew Strathern. 1999c. Female spirit cults as a window on gender relations in the highlands of Papua New Guinea. *Journal of the Royal Anthropological Institute* 5(3):345–360.

Stewart, Pamela J., and Andrew Strathern. 1999d.Time at the end: The highlands of Papua New Guinea. In Christin Kocher-Schmid, ed., *Expecting the Day of Wrath: Versions of the Millennium in Papua New Guinea,* pp. 131–144. Port Moresby, Papua New Guinea: National Research Institute.

Stewart, Pamela J., and Andrew Strathern. 2000. Naming places: Duna evocations of landscape in Papua New Guinea. *People and Culture in Oceania.* Vol. 16:87–107.

Strathern, A. 1971. *The Rope of Moka.* Cambridge: Cambridge University Press.

Strathern, A. 1974. Kinship, descent and locality: Some New Guinea examples. In Jack Goody, ed., *The Character of Kinship*, pp. 21–33. Cambridge: Cambridge University Press.

Strathern, A. 1975. Why is shame on the skin? *Ethnology* 14(4): 347–356.

Strathern, A. 1982. Witchcraft, greed, cannibalism and death. In Maurice Bloch and Jonathan Parry eds., *Death and the Regeneration of Life*, pp. 111–133. Cambridge: Cambridge University Press.

Strathern, A. 1996. *Body Thoughts.* Ann Arbor: University of Michigan Press.

Strathern, Andrew, and Pamela J. Stewart. 1997. Ballads as popular performance art in Papua New Guinea and Scotland. Discussion Papers Series, no. 2, pp.

1–17. Townsville, Queensland: James Cook University, Centre for Pacific Studies.

Strathern, Andrew, and Pamela J. Stewart. 1999. *Curing and Healing: Medical Anthropology in Global Perspective.* Durham, NC: Carolina Academic Press.

Strathern, Andrew and Pamela J. Stewart. 2000a. *Arrow Talk: Transaction, Transition, and Contradiction in New Guinea Highlands History.* Kent, Ohio: Kent State University Press.

Strathern, Andrew, and Pamela J. Stewart. 2000b. *The Python's Back: Pathways of Comparison Between Indonesia and Melanesia.* Westport, CT: Bergin and Garvey.

Tuzin, Donald. 1997. *The Cassowary's Revenge: The Life and Death of Masculinity in a New Guinea Society.* Chicago: University of Chicago Press.

Wagner, Roy. 1991. The fractal person. In Maurice Godelier and Marilyn Strathern, eds., *Big Men and Great Men*, pp. 159–173. Cambridge: Cambridge University Press.

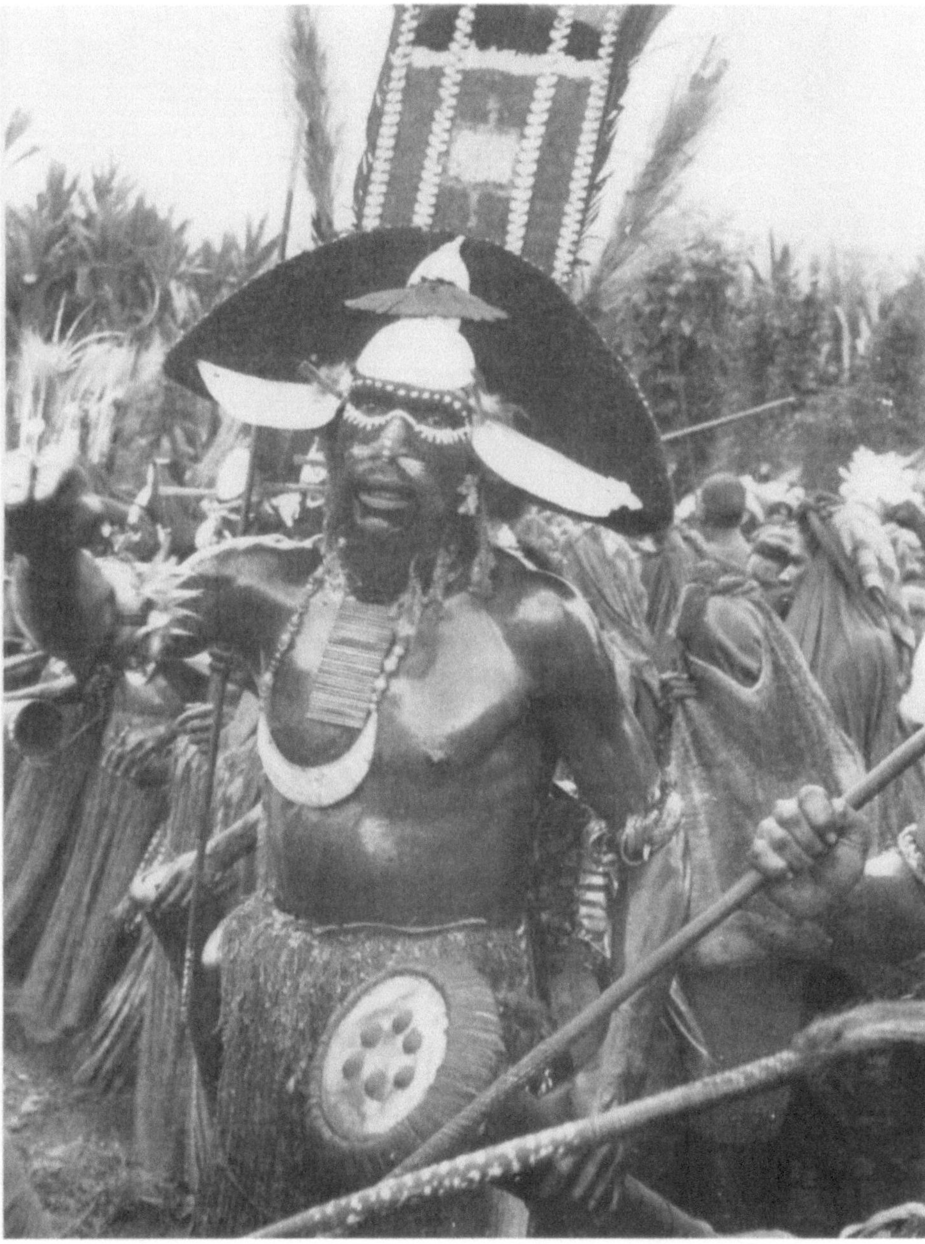

Dancer at a *moka* (exchange ceremony) among the Mundika people at Klönd near Tomba in 1969. The dancer's body is liberally oiled to give the skin a shining, healthy appearance. His large, horned wig is made from human hair, evidence of the hair's power of growth.

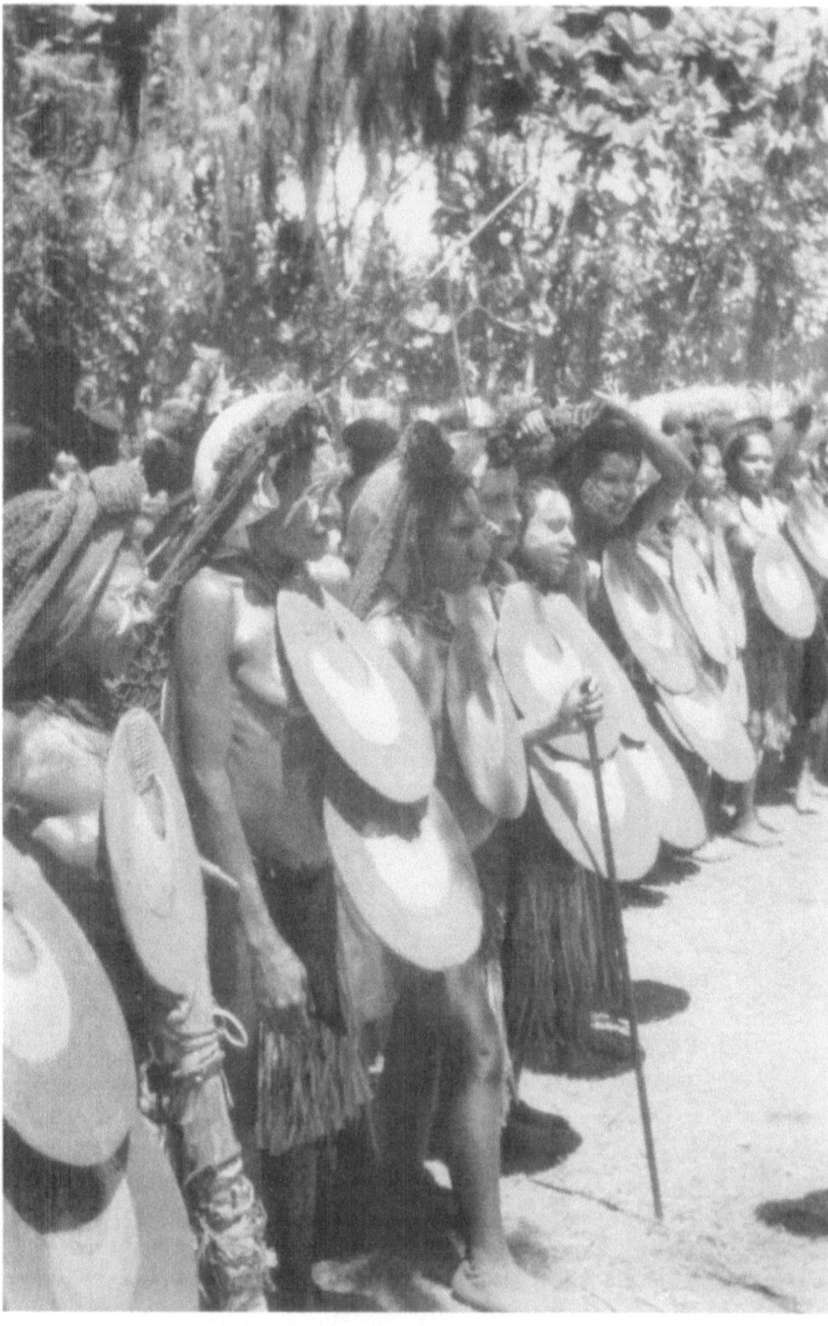

Women dancers at a *moka* (exchange ceremony) of the Mundika people near Tomba in 1969. Their bodies are adorned with large pearl shells, which are indicative of wealth and well-being.

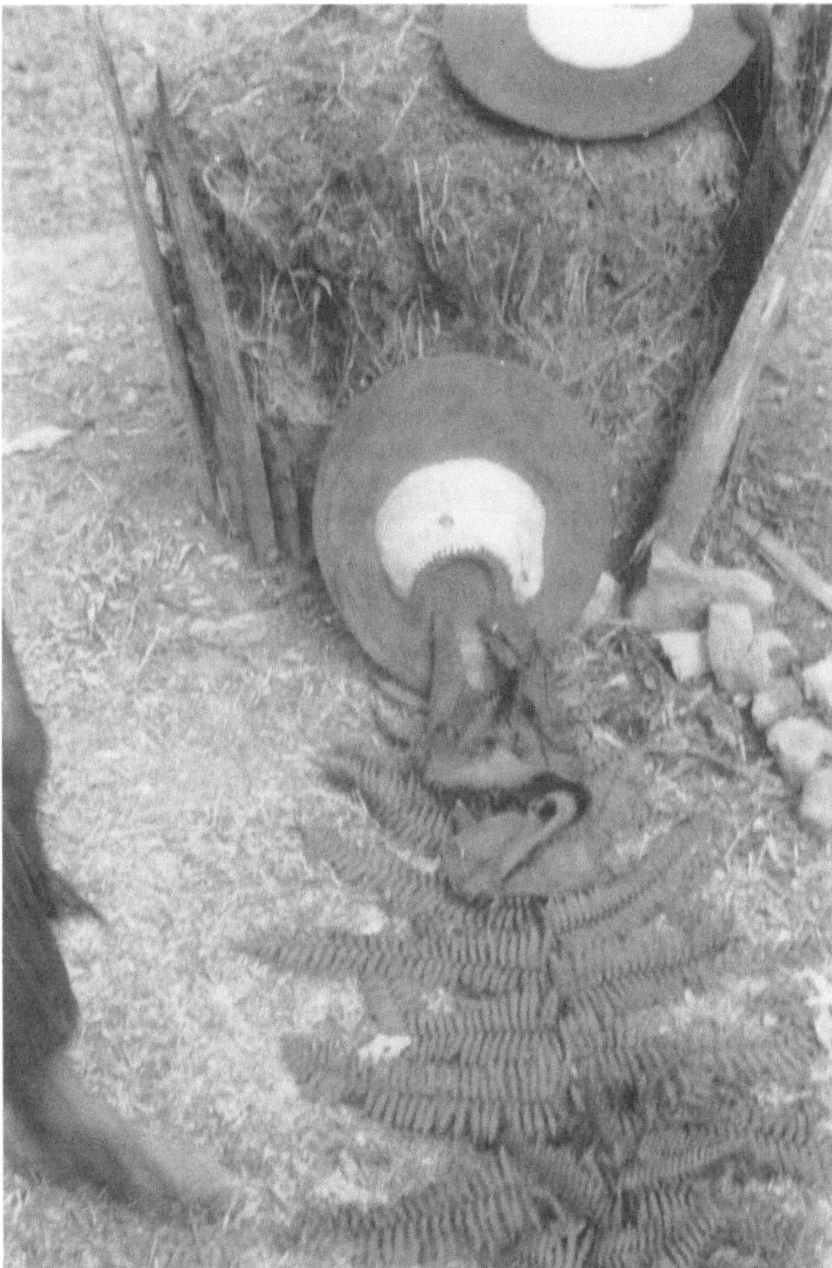

An especially fine pearl shell, mounted on a resin board and painted with red ocher, propped up beside an old ceremonial tub at the head of a dancing ground (1970s). The shell's glistening yellow color evinces its character as a kind of healthy skin similar to that of the human body.

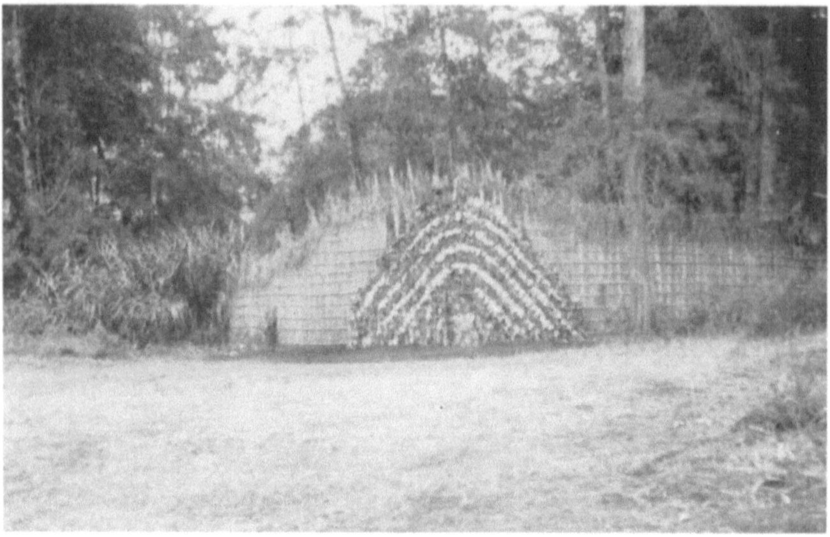

The main fence in front of a Wöp cult site, with an elaborate decoration of brown and silver-colored leaves over the gateway, Nebilyer Valley, 1965 (Kulir area).

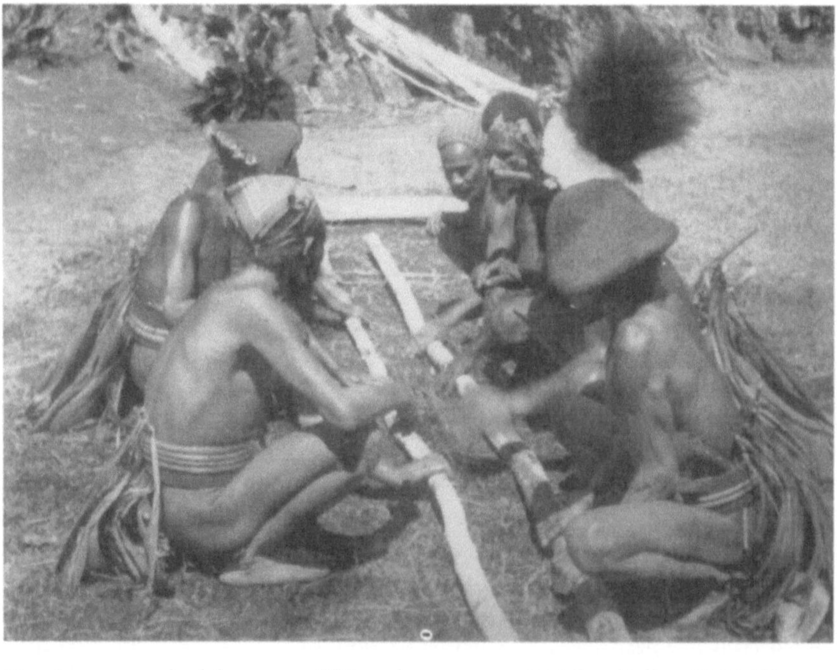

Ritual experts and celebrants at a Wöp cult, ceremony, Nebilyer Valley, 1965. They are holding lengths of *wantep* (*Trema amboinensis*) wood that will be sung about in a spell for growth (Kulir area).

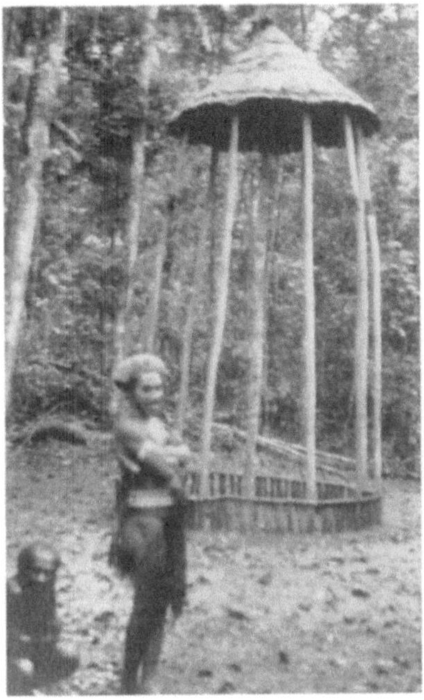

A tower house for a Wöp cult performance, Nebilyer Valley, August 1965.

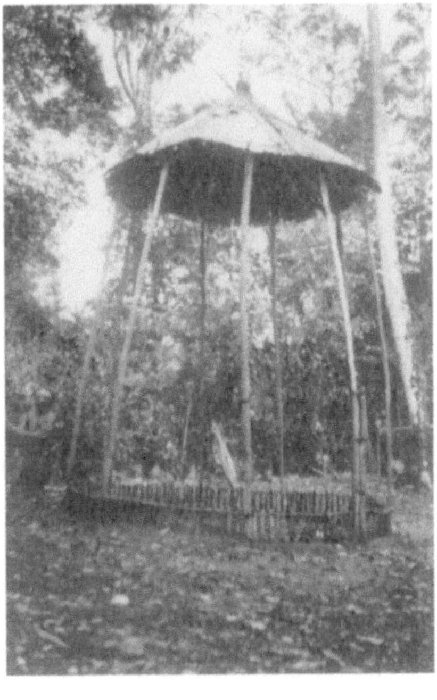

A tower house for a Wöp cult performance, Nebilyer Valley, 1965.

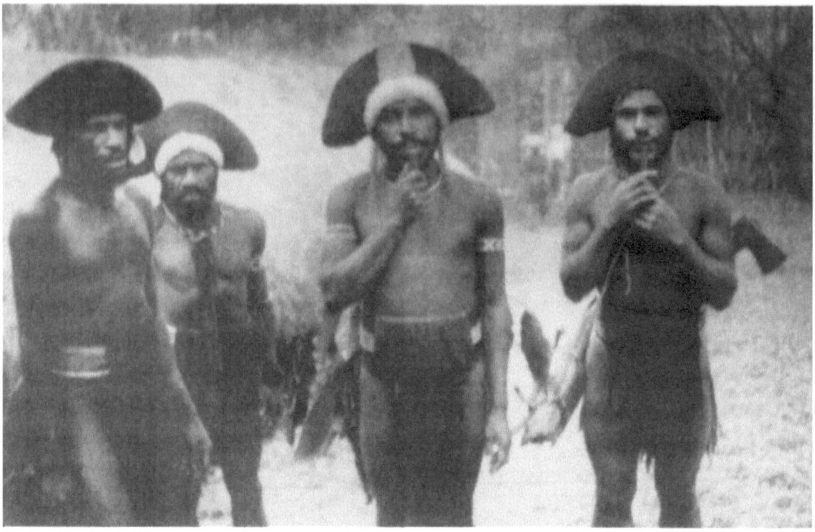

Young initiates beside the food-roasting house for the Wöp cult, Nebilyer Valley, 1965. Two are blowing small whistles to warn noninitiates to stay out of the way when materials for the cult are brought in (Kulir area).

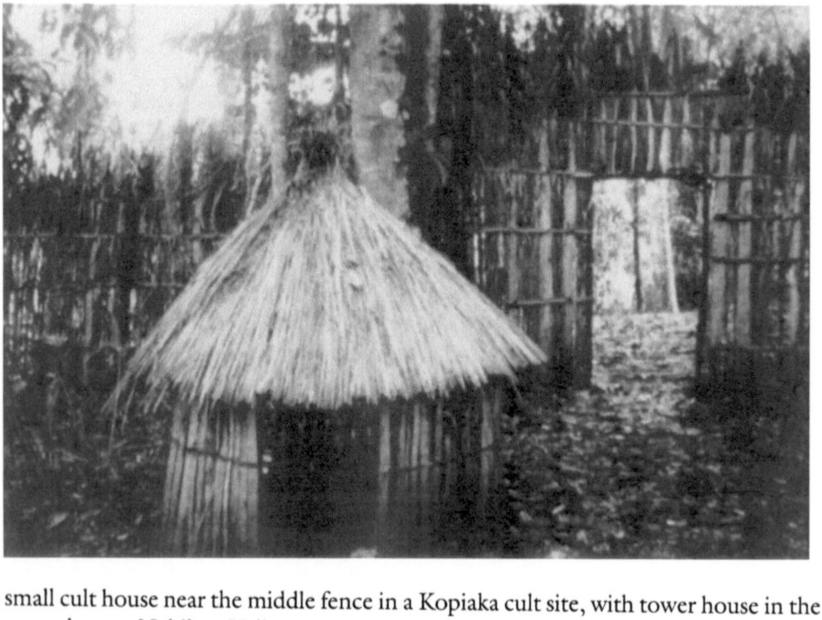

A small cult house near the middle fence in a Kopiaka cult site, with tower house in the next enclosure, Nebilyer Valley, 1965.

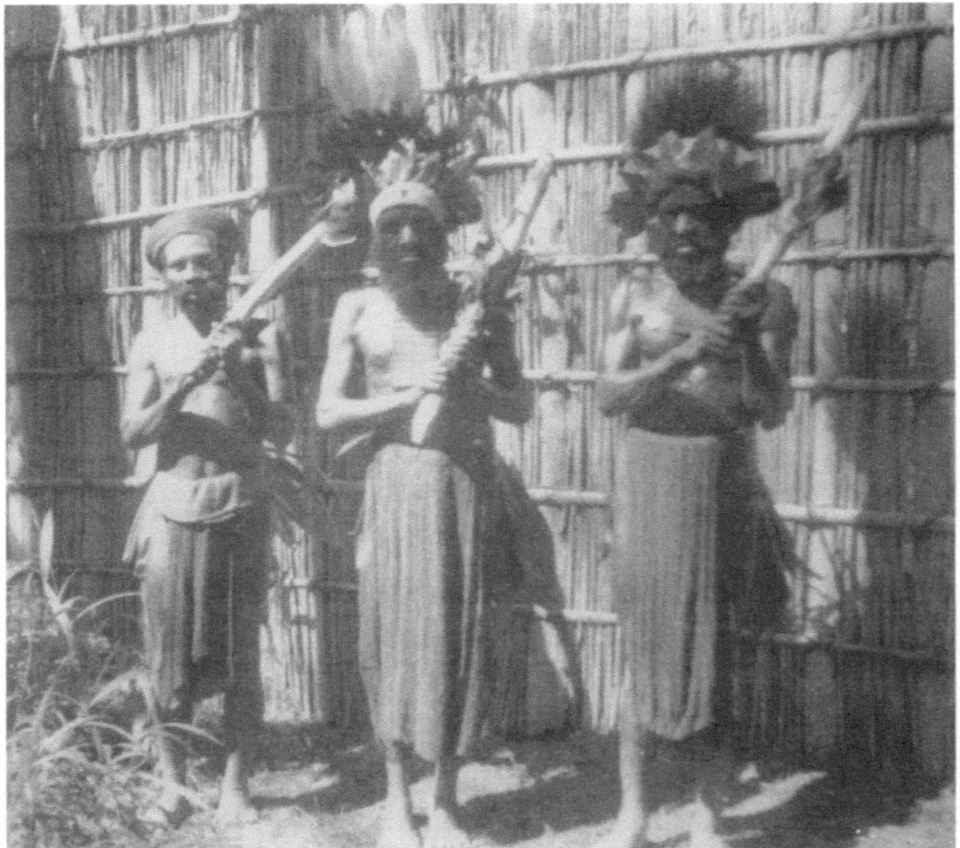

Three ritual experts for the Wöp cult line up at the fence of the cult area with clubs, ready to sacrifice pigs (Kulir area).

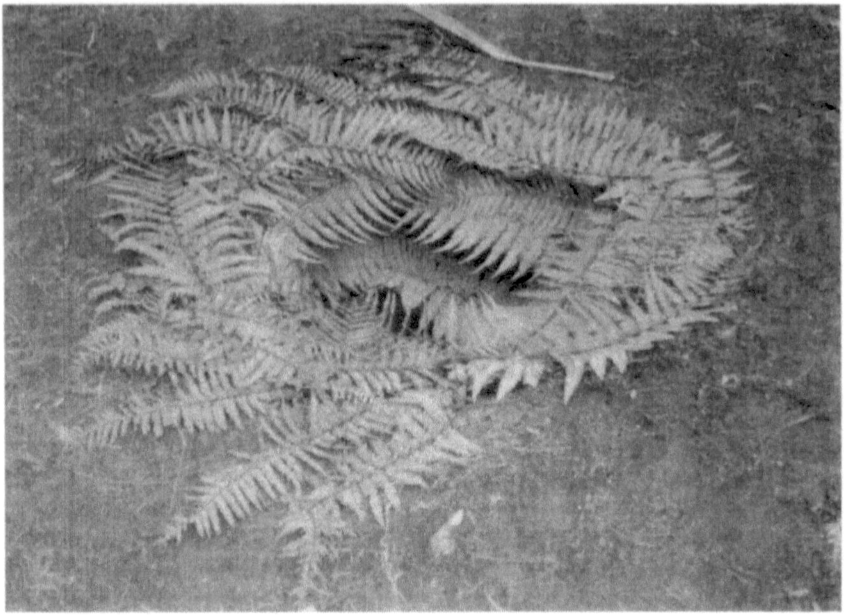

*Nöng* ferns carefully spread to cover a spring source, the "eye" of the Wöp spirit, Nebilyer Valley, 1965 (Kulir area).

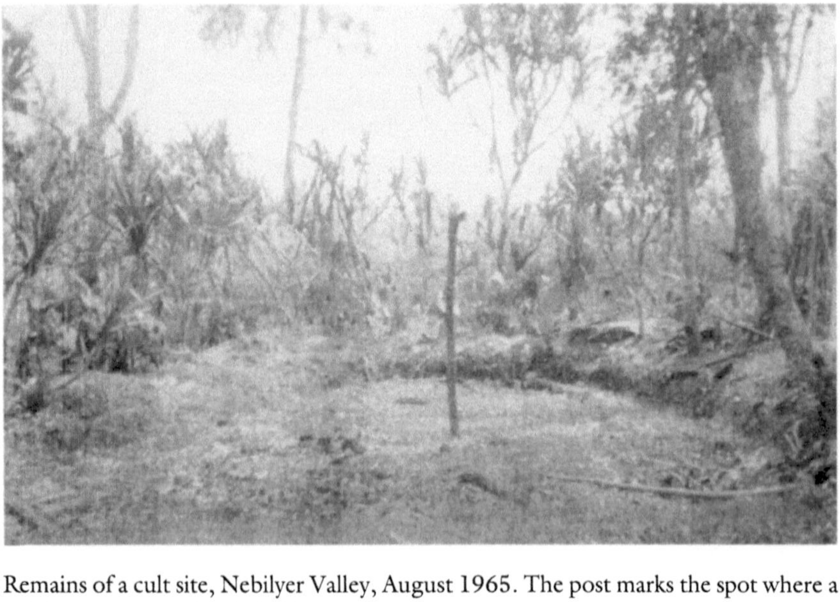

Remains of a cult site, Nebilyer Valley, August 1965. The post marks the spot where a cult house was previously built.

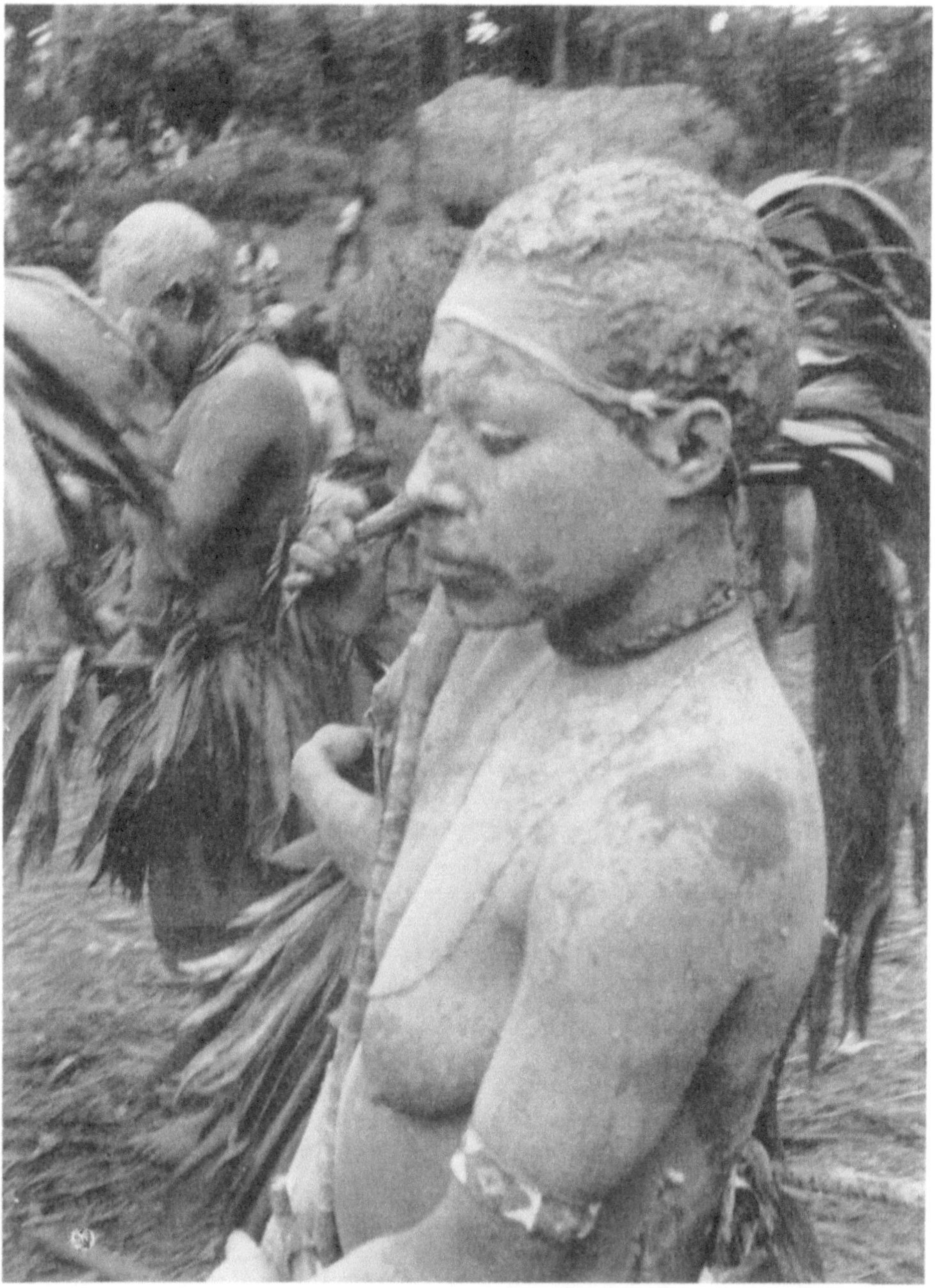

Female mourner among the Ndika people near Mount Hagen, early 1970s. Her hair, face, and body are plastered with white mourning clay, and she carries a cordyline switch. Earth paints are used to mark the body in particular ways (for healing, grief, or celebration, for example), and act to produce a kind of second skin on the person that intimately connects the human body to the ground.

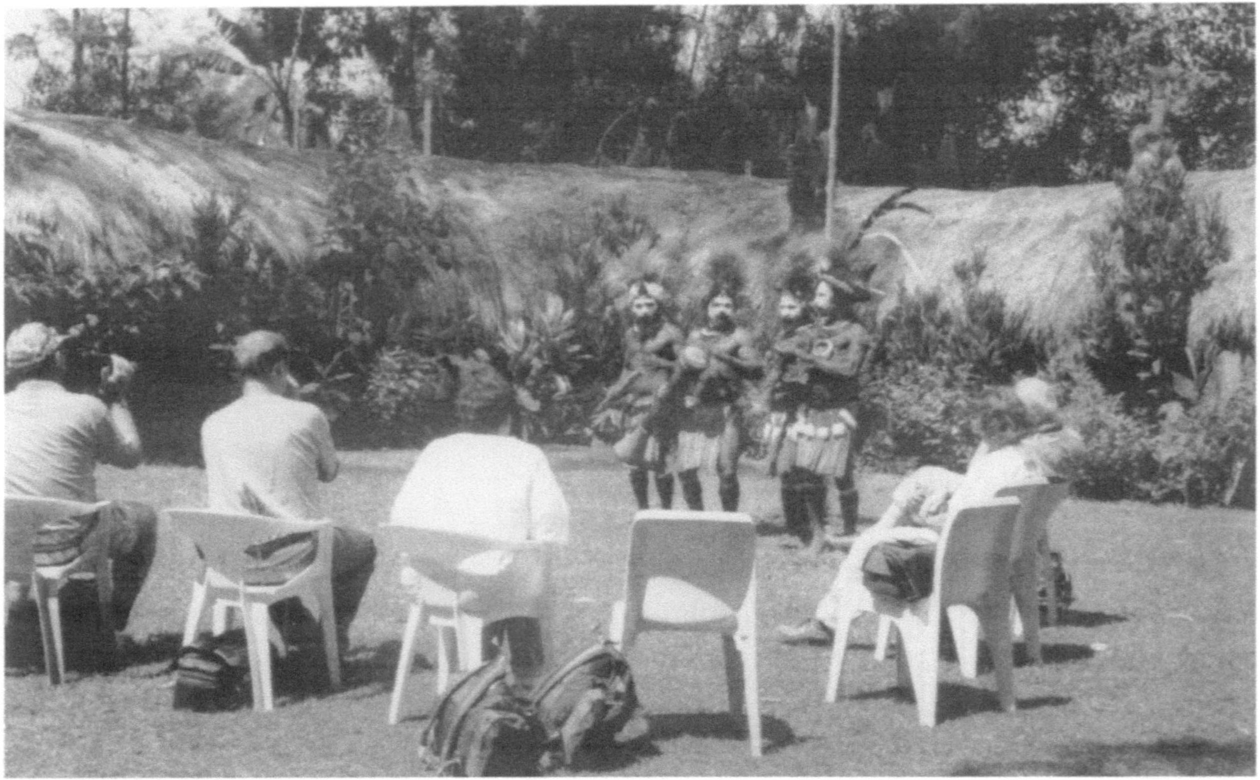

German tourists at a hotel in Mount Hagen take photographs of four decorated men from the Huli area, Southern Highlands Province. (The Huli area is culturally similar to that of the Duna). Tourist displays have for the most part replaced indigenous dance contexts as venues for obtaining money as well as displaying a healthy appearance.

# CHAPTER 5

# Substance Transfer: Conception, Growth, and Nurturance in Highlands Papua New Guinea

*Pamela J. Stewart and Andrew Strathern*

## RITUALS TO SEEK FERTILITY

Ritual practices in the Highlands of Papua New Guinea had growth and fertility as one of their major aims. In many instances fertility was envisioned in terms of the female and male fluids that lead to conception and growth. Ritual practices were performed to ensure that the proper placement of these fluids was maintained and that gendered bodies were properly developed or grown in order for society to remain in balance with the cosmos and to sustain the perpetuation of the clan group (Stewart 1998; Stewart and Strathern 1999a; Meigs 1984; Sillitoe 1985, 1996; Wiessner and Tumu 1998).

In the Hagen, Pangia, and Duna areas of Papua New Guinea, concerns with fertility found their expression in a number of rituals (Strathern and Stewart 1998a, 2000). In Hagen the Amb Kor (Female Spirit) ritual was held periodically to ensure that women would bear children and that the fertility of the ground as well as of the livestock (pigs) would continue. The ritual also aimed at ridding the community of sickness that ultimately impaired fertility. If these ritual practices were carried out properly, the Amb Kor would place part of her fertility powers in the cult stones that the male ritual performers had gathered as repositories into which her powers could flow and be retained. These stones were surrounded by cool ferns and anointed with pork fat (*kng kopong*, symbolizing semen) and red ocher (*ui kela*, symbolizing blood), then buried in the local soil of the group at the conclusion of the cult ritual performance (Strathern and Stewart 1998a; Stewart 1998). The cult stones possess fertility power, as eggs do. Meggitt (1965:107) reports that the Mae Enga describe certain sacred stones as "eggs of the Sun." The Pangia people referred to the cult stones (*tapa mu*) used in the *tapa* (male) cult as "eggs" or "testicles" of the *tapa* spirit (Stewart and Strathern 1999b).

Among the Duna there are stones known as *auwi* (sacred) stones. These are thought to be the petrified heart or some other internal part of ancestors that after a number of generations reveal themselves to a descendant. A special ritual must be performed when these stones "show" themselves to the descendants, otherwise sickness or death may ensue.

The association of stones with fertility and healing power among the Duna (and elsewhere) depends on an overall model of transformation between elements of the cosmos, to the effect that the life-giving element of water may be transformed into fat or juice, and this in turn into stone. Thus, in myths regarding the Female Spirit in the Duna area, the Spirit is connected with rainstorms and floods, and also with round pools through which people travel to reach the land of the dead. She also can manifest herself in a kind of marsupial, which if trapped contains in its stomach special stone crystals that are used in magic to make the skin of unmarried men good, with healthy fat just below the surface. Finally, she may enter into cult stones such as prehistoric mortars, making these her "house," so that they form a focus for her cult.

In the past, crystals like those found in the marsupial's stomach were used in Hagen as magic items to make pigs grow. They form in caves where water collects or where an underground stream finds its way. Such crystals can be seen as solidified forms of life force akin to the fat that develops under the skin of pigs, and is called "water" by the Duna.

The same magical life force can be carried in wind and smoke. When the Duna Female Spirit shows herself to the ritual bachelor who presides over the boys' growth cult and comes to him as his "wife," she appears with lightning, a rainstorm, and floodwater, accompanied by the cries of pigs and children. She gives power to the smoke that billows up from fires that the cult neophytes light before their emergence from their enclosure. As the smoke reaches the nostrils of marriageable girls, they begin to think of the youths and desire them. The spells for the boys' growth prominently mention the power of water to make them grow, contributing to their flesh and to the volume of their head hair, which the ritual expert teases out for them.

The Hagen Amb Kor (Female Spirit) similarly has a multiple set of manifestations: she, too, appears in lighting and rain, but also as menstrual blood, in human form as a bride, and finally in the shape of her cult stones that are anointed and buried in the ground. In other words, she can appear in the most fluid and volatile of ways, in the "solid" form of a person, and in the "most solid" form as a stone. These images therefore express a dialectic of fluidity and fixity of power, and the cult stones represent a collectivized fixity of power as a transform of individualized fluidity. This conclusion clearly holds for both the Hagen and the Duna cases.

The theme of stones as repositories of fertility powers is a common one in Papua New Guinea (see, e.g., the extensive literature survey by Riesenfeld 1950). Here we give a few more examples to illustrate the following points: (1) cult stones are seen as repositories not just of power, but also of powers of fertility and growth; (2) they represent a solidification of these powers that in other manifestations may be seen as fluid; and (3) such stones accordingly are not seen as inert objects but as living beings. We include below one case from Borneo that clearly demonstrates point (2), even though it belongs to Indonesia, not Melanesia (see also Strathern and Stewart 2000).

Brigitta Hauser-Schäublin (1995) describes a ritual practice among Abelam males of the Middle Sepik of Papua New Guinea, who keep oddly shaped stones in their yam houses that are thought to promote growth and fertility of yams and these stones are sometimes buried in the yam gardens. In addition to these personally owned stones, the community retains a few stones that are kept in a special hut, access to which is restricted to one or two designated men. These stones are associated with the growth of major tuber crops, and prior to planting time the stone(s) are decorated, *like a long yam* and *like a ceremonial dancer*. Growers who hope to grow outstanding long yams send shell rings to the stone, which are placed directionally so as to act "as a *bridge* that carries the stone's power" toward the grower's garden. Hauser-Schäublin suggests that these stones, which are "the symbol of men's procreative powers over vegetable life," are equated with menarcheal girls, who are the symbols of women's procreative powers. "Both are secluded in special huts surrounded by gender-specific secrecy. . . . Both are ritually washed with the same mixture of herbs and cane juice before their ceremonial decoration. . . . Both are kept hidden and never brought to the ceremonial grounds, feasts to honor both are held" (pp. 45–46). The ritual painting and burial of these stones is reminiscent of how the Hagen Amb Kor stones are treated.

Another example of how stones are used as receptacles of fertility powers is the *barasi dirukui* ritual from the Zogari village on Manam Island, Papua New Guinea, described by Nancy Lutkehaus (1995). The *barasi dirukui* is an annual ceremony aiming to renew the ground's fertility and safeguard the good health and prosperity of the villagers. "As part of the *barasi* celebration, boys and girls are beaten ritually, and a set of stones, known as *barasi* stones [stones with holes in them, representing female fertility], are ritually washed" (p. 201). These ritual activities resemble cultural themes that occur in female first menstruation rites and male initiation into the community. "The stones are first washed . . . then smeared with the red pigment known as taro, an act symbolically analogous to washing and painting a young girl for her *imoaziri* [puberty] rites and marriage" (p. 201). This treatment of the stones is similar to the preparation of the Hagen Amb Kor stones, which were smeared with red ocher and pig grease (*kopong*) prior to their burial in the ground, where they were meant to enhance fertility.

Parallels and contrasts to the cultural knowledge regarding the Amb Kor stones can further be found in Jay Bernstein's (1997) study of spirit stones and shamanism among the Taman of Borneo. Bernstein's title, *Spirits Captured in Stone*, itself captures an important element in the ethnoaesthetics of movement and power that seems fundamental to such a comparison. In the Taman case, participants in a ritual to establish a new shaman (*balien*) play music to attract spirits and then capture these spirits by tapping dishes with special leaves until stones appear in them. The stones are said to be soft at first appearance and to be hardened by the application of cooking oil, after which they become black and glossy. At the end of a long, repeated process of capturing stones in this way, the shamanic adept is expected to catch his or her own stone, which will become a repository for power. The ability to find such stones is said to come from dreams, as happens with the Amb Kor in Hagen, and the stones must be fed with rice and palm wine in order to keep them with their human possessors.

Here, we wish to draw out the significance of "capturing in stone." The basic trope is that of transforming fluidity into solidity, paradigmatic of the creation of identity in general. As long as a spirit is shadowy and unseen, it cannot be brought under the fixed control of an adept. Once it has become stone or entered into a stone, its transformation into a beneficial force has begun. The same sequence appears in the Amb Kor. A potential adept or cult sponsor dreams of the Spirit in conjunction with sicknesses arising in the dreamer's group. Later the adept finds the Spirit in stone form and sets up the cult site; the ritual effects not only a curing of sicknesses but also the enhancement of fertility and health in general.

The Mararoko women of the Kewa-speaking area in the Southern Highlands Province of Papua New Guinea have similar types of healing stones called *lugogo*, which they use when their husbands or children fall ill. The stones are heated along with other stones in an earth oven in which special foods are cooked. These foods are eaten not by the sick person but by the wife/mother on behalf of her husband or children. The use of these stones in this manner is a reversal of the gendered role that the husband would have filled in the past, when he would have participated in spirit cults to secure the health and fertility of his family (MacDonald 1991:140). In this process the innate power of the stones is tapped, and there is no direct interaction with a particular spirit whose temperament must be delicately handled in order to ensure a beneficent response.

This is unlike the relationship between a spirit and a *balien* adept in Taman, where the force of the spirit must be tamed and made beneficent. This interaction in the Taman case can be seen as a sexual one, as can the relationship of the Amb Kor cult adherents in Hagen with the Female Spirit, who is said to come as a bride to the man who dreams of her and finds her stone. In fact, upon finding an Amb Kor stone, a man will often say that he has found his wife. After initiation, the *balien* is required to pay a fine to his or her spouse, in recognition of the fact that the spirit has "violated" their marriage. Over time the *balien* acquires a complete set of spirit (*tamang*) stones, each representing a member of the kindred, and the stones individually announce their identities to the novice *balien* in dreams. These ideas represent a development of notions found also in the Amb Kor context in Hagen, but are taken to a point of specialized appropriation by a single adept who becomes a shaman.

The basic tropes of power, however, are the same in both cases. Stones are "good to think with" in this context because they represent a solidification of the fluidity of power. This is in accordance with the idea in Highlands New Guinea that the amount of spirit power a stone has is assessed in terms of the stone's *weight* in relation to its size. In the Taman case, spirit stones belong absolutely to an individual shaman, and they cannot be exchanged or inherited, although they can be used by another shaman. In the case of Hagen Amb Kor stones, cult performers should find their own stones, as revealed to them by the Spirit, and these stones should then be buried in the ground and also never exchanged further.

Beatrice Blackwood (1935), in her work on Buka, then a part of the mandated Territory of New Guinea, discusses a series of natural rocks or stones that were thought of as *urar* spirits. Stone and spirit were "completely identified, so that the *urar* is the stone." At night it might assume human form and go fishing or dancing (Blackwood 1935:527). Blackwood also describes a number of upright stone pillars, some incised, credited with the ability to grow in size, to make people sick, or to resist being stolen. Such stones were spoken of as kin to their owners. They might be washed and anointed in rituals, bathed with pig's blood or painted with red ocher. In one case boys were taken to the stone and their skins were cicatrized before it. The stones were sometimes incised with designs like those of cicatrization, and Blackwood suggests that this was purposive. Cicatrization was supposed to help children to grow, to make persons attractive to the opposite sex, and to make milk flow in young women's breasts (p. 538). Blackwood argues that the stones were held to conduce to those same ends, and that they "may perhaps have formed part of an elaborate fertility ritual" (p. 540).

MacDonald (1991) describes how the cult stones for the *ribu* fertility and wealth cult were used by the Mararoko Kewa of Papua New Guinea:

> First the stones, which were kept buried in the tall spirit house were unearthed and rubbed with possum fur by a cult leader. There was at least one stone for each of the *repa* [family group] represented in the men's house. Then pigs would be killed. . . . After the pigs had been killed their throats would be slit and blood smeared over the stones. Red earth, various oils, pig fat and animal faeces could also be applied to the stones to create different markings. People say that the ghosts ate the blood and fat of the pigs (p. 136).

Another cult ritual that MacDonald mentions as still being performed in the 1980s by the Mararoko was for the *keveta pamo* (stone woman) cult; this particularly focused on ensuring the fertility of women and pigs (p. 139). Here we see the spirit being referred to as a stone, the object that often serves as the vessel in which these powerful spirits dwell.

The Konda Dani of Irian Jaya used polished stones in rituals to enhance garden fertility and to make pigs grow well (O'Brien 1970:38). They used another set of longer polished stones called *jao* as part of bride-price payments and indemnity payments. *Jao* came in two shapes: narrow, rounded ones and flat ones that were slightly longer and wider than the first type (pp. 38, 408). Their color ranged from dark green to blue (p. 337). Among the Grand Valley Dani the flat stones frequently were adorned with a covering similar to the skirts worn by women (O'Brien 1970:337–338, citing Bromley 1965:21). The Konda Dani did not decorate their stones in this way, but the men would rub grease into them while relaxing in the communal men's house.

> *Jao* stones are displayed as part of marriage payments, male spectators spend a great deal of time arranging and rearranging them, and rubbing them with pig grease. Ideally, there should be an equal number of male [i.e. the narrow, rounded stones in O'Brien's usage] and female [i.e., the flat stones in O'Brien's usage] stones in any marriage payment, so that the stones can be laid out in pairs with the male stone resting on the female stone. The Dani are explicit in stating that such an arrangement of paired stones represents human sexual intercourse and that the bride and groom should emulate the *jao*. Men also say that fondling the stones and rubbing them with pig fat reminds them of copulation. (O'Brien 1970:338)

O'Brien (pp. 338–339) quotes Ploeg (1962, personal communication) as stating that the Dani at Bokondini "told him [Ploeg] that the first such stone [*jao*] was used to stop the bleeding of a child's umbilical cord and *jao* were then introduced into the marriage ceremonies."

The link between marriage and fertility is also highlighted by the Hagen Female Spirit, who was seen as coming inside the clan group as a bride to the men, who would honor her during the cult ritual, while bringing fertility to the cult participants' human wives. The burying of her stones in the soil of the clan physically represented the part of the Spirit that stayed within the clan boundaries after the ritual even as the Spirit herself moved on, as an out-marrying sister/daughter would move out from the group, to the next group, who would receive her as a bride and accept her gifts of fertility. Thus a part of the Spirit and the substance of hers that was within her stones stayed with one group while a part of her substantiality traveled to another group. This is analogous to the situation of human women who marry into a group, bringing their fertility powers with them, and then their daughters subsequently carry fertility to other groups, thereby establishing alliances. Each man who participated in the cult ritual performance, and by extension his family, hoped to benefit from the Spirit's fertility gifts. The enhanced ability of wives to produce sons was especially sought from the Female Spirit, so as to build and strengthen the local group.

The Amb Kor is just one example of a series of Female Spirits found in the Highlands of New Guinea who were looked to as sources of fertility (Stewart and Strathern 1998a). In Pangia the local Female Spirit was called Laiyeroa or Aroa Ipono; in Duna she was known as Payame Ima. In addition to the rituals of these Female Spirit cults other fertility rituals were practiced that involved the presentation of bodily substances to spirits living within the ground. In the Duna area *hambua hatya* was a ritual that took place along an extended trackway between the parish of Yokona, near the Strickland River and Lake Kopiago, and a sacred site located far to the south near to the territory of the Huli people, called Kelokili. The ritual putatively involved the sacrifice and dismemberment of a male who had proven his fertility by siring children. Parts of a victim's body were said to have been buried at specific cult spots (Stewart 1998).

Another fertility ritual from the Duna area that involved the movement of body parts along a trackway between the Strickland River and Kelokili was the *kirao hatya*. In this ritual, menstrual blood was collected from a virgin of a particular descent group and was carried in a sealed bamboo tube along the trackway to Kelokili, where it was placed in a hole in the earth, appeasing the male spirit who lived there (Strathern and Stewart 1998a). The woman who donated her menstrual blood had shown her reproductive potential through the onset of menstruation. After her blood was placed in the earth, the donor was expected to remain a virgin and was known as Auwi Ima (Sacred Woman). All of these rituals symbolically or physically embedded fertility-producing substances/powers into the earth so as to bring progeny to humans and animals, and to renew the ground so that crops would grow well and food would be plentiful.

Fertility rituals were historically imported into the Hagen and Pangia areas with a set of ideas about how gender relations should be structured. In both Pangia and Hagen the Female Spirit cults were a means not just of bringing fertility but also of providing protection to men against the potentially lethal powers of menstrual blood that was out of its "proper" place. Menstruation in a female signals the onset of her reproductive potential, and in a sexually active, fertile female the absence of menstrual flow is a sign that the procreative act has begun within her body. But for a man it was thought that menstrual blood could produce sickness and even death if taken in through the penis or through the mouth by ingestion of contaminated food. Thus, women were segregated from men into special menstrual huts where they cooked their own food and did not prepare food for their spouse or male relations during their menstrual flow. Interestingly, in Pangia it was thought that if menstrual blood did come into a man, it could produce an ectopic pregnancy that would eventuate in death because of the lack of a uterus and vagina to expel the fetus from the body (Stewart and Strathern 1999a).

Meigs and others have noted other examples of fears of "ectopic pregnancy" in males (Hayano 1974 [cited in Meigs 1984]; Glick 1963:117; Williams 1969:201–202). Meigs tells us that among the Hua people of Eastern

Highland Province of Papua New Guinea, "male pregnancy is presented without excuse or qualification as a dangerous outcome of improper practice. Some informants even claim to have seen fetuses after their removal from men's bodies, an operation performed by non–Hua specialists" (Meigs 1984:47–48). Williams (1969:201–202) gives an example of the Keraki of the Trans-Fly area, who used lime as a "contraceptive" so as "to ensure that young men do not become pregnant." In this example it is thought that "male pregnancy" can arise from sexual intercourse between men. Thus the agent of conception in men is seen as semen, as opposed to female blood, among the Keraki.

Comparisons are often made between substances of the earth and substances in the human body. The earth paints used in self-decoration often carry associations of this sort. Red ocher, for example, a favorite substance both for body decoration and for the painting of stones, is clearly related to blood. Earths used in curing and protective magic are seen as having cooling properties, and may be yellow or white. One element that has particular significance for the Duna people is ash from wood fires. They are aware that ash from fires burned when clearing gardens increases the fertility of soil. Their myths also record a cataclysmic period when ash fell from the sky and choked the land and its streams, after which, however, fertility was renewed (see Frankel 1986 for similar ideas explicitly linked to renewal among the Huli; see also Biersack 1995). A dead person's spirit or *tini* could be encapsulated in the charcoal and ashes from wood used to heat the stones for the earth ovens made for a funeral feast, and the spirit-ash could then be transported in a special container back to the dead person's natal area if he or she had died elsewhere. A male forest spirit, the *tsiri*, was known to throw ashes at people who intruded on his domain. Although this action was aggressive, the *tsiri* was also pelting people with a fertility-bearing substance, and if he was placated by sacrifices, he also could confer benefits such as pig and cowrie shell wealth. The ash from the singed hair of a marsupial could be spread on sweet potatoes fed to pigs, to help the pigs grow well. All of these examples show a connection between ash as residue and ash as a fertility-giving substance among the Duna.

## CONCEPTION AND INTRAUTERINE GROWTH

In Hagen, when a woman becomes pregnant, conception is described as an event that involves the mixing of the sexual *kopong* (grease) of the female (vaginal fluids) and that of the male (semen) as a first step. This is followed by the male *kopong* surrounding the *mema* (blood) of the female to produce a fetal packet like an egg (*köi mukl*), described as *kum ronom*, "it wraps." This packet will become a child if nurtured in the womb (Strathern and Stewart 1998b). This embodied sequence of actions is paralleled by the burying of the grease- (*kopong*) and ocher- (symbolic of *mema*) smeared stones at the conclusion of the Amb Kor Female Spirit cult ritual, detailed above.

Some of the Hageners realize that during pregnancy the child grows and becomes bigger, and that special foods must be eaten by the mother to ensure the health of the growing child. It is clear from the narratives given below that the *kopong* (grease) and the *mema* (blood) of the female sustain and nurture the developing child in utero. The category of *kopong* includes the nurturant quality of foods that are especially eaten during pregnancy, such as greens, other juicy vegetable foods, and pork fat. Also, red foods are thought to help to replenish the blood and are eaten at this time. Male *kopong* (semen) is thought to be deleterious during the period of breast-feeding because it is believed to "spoil" breast milk, and therefore to be harmful to the growth of a child. Hence there is a taboo on intercourse during postpartum breast-feeding years.

Glimpses of detailed views on conception and nurturance are provided in two interviews, one with a senior man named Wömndi in 1979 (Chapter 7), and the other with the female ritual expert we have called Anita, in 1998 (Chapter 4).

Wömndi introduces a number of complexities into the picture. First, he points out that God is involved in conception, slotting God in where the ghosts of dead kin traditionally appear. Second, he suggests that some women become pregnant more readily than others because inside them they have two things like beans that stand up, an image that sounds somewhat like a description of ovaries. Third, he directly links semen, spinal fluid, and head substance while also arguing that the head substance (*peng konya*) plays a role in judgment or thought processes. Finally, he sees a role for the "grease" (*kopong*) of both male and female in the formation of the child's body. Females especially supply blood, but they also supply their own grease. Wömndi does not take up the question of nurturance in utero, however.

Anita (see chapter 4) knew magic to induce pregnancy, to facilitate birthing, and to make children grow big and strong. For fertility she collected water from a stream in a bamboo tube and bespelled it, then gave it to the patient to drink. She collected fresh leaves from riverbanks and made them into magic food for the woman to eat. In her spells she called on three things: water pools, eels, and the eggs of a particular flightless bird. Pools with their water flowing around represent the idea of the child being formed and coming out; eels are slippery, and so the child will slip out easily; chicks inside the bird's eggs break their shells open with their beaks and come out quickly. The spell functioned equally for pregnancy itself and for an easy birth. Anita also massaged the stomach of a woman about to give birth, using cool riverbank leaves to make the body "cool and fresh" (*kundil*) so that the child would emerge.

Anita, no doubt, influenced by Catholic teachings, declared that God puts the baby inside the pregnant woman and feeds it, making it grow. She did not have a specific theory of how the fetus feeds or grows beyond this attribution to God and his power. Nevertheless, she clearly thought that the blood and grease of both the father and the mother go into the child and make its body; and because the bodies of people require food in order to keep their blood and other substances healthy, the implication is that the fetus also requires food in order to grow and be healthy. Tying off the navel string prevents the nourishing blood from flowing out of the infant, so the umbilical cord is the obvious candidate for being the conduit along which nourishing agency flows into the womb.

One of our Hagen collaborators (Mr. Ru-Kundil), who is a local specialist on traditional knowledge, described the process of growth that occurs during gestation in utero as follows:

> It was previously thought [i.e. before health care workers told Hageners otherwise] that a woman had two cords inside of herself that fed into the growing child. One cord was a path for the woman's blood to flow into the child [the umbilicus] and the other went to her breast and carried her milk to the growing child.

Though not all Hageners described this two-cord nurturance system, all spoke of the mother's blood carrying growth-sustaining fluids derived from the foods that she ate during her pregnancy. The mother is therefore definitely seen as more than just a vessel or container for the child; she is also a source of nurturance and growth. The vital significance of the umbilical cord as a source of nurturance is further built on in traditional practices that followed a birth. The father of the child was supposed to build a small fence or enclosure within which a cordyline or a banana tree would be planted. The navel cord and the afterbirth would be buried in the enclosure. The child's feces could also be thrown inside it. These were seen as nourishing the plant. As the plant was rooted in the soil, so would the child be attached to the locality. It is interesting in this regard to note that the plant fed on a part of the child's *maternal* substance as well as on the normatively *paternal* soil (i.e., the clan land of the father). The child thus continued to be seen as a product of both paternal and maternal substance, and the latter was localized, as it were, within a paternal territory as a *mbo*, a shoot or stock. Children of the same mother or of sisters are spoken of as *wamb tam tenda*, people of the same navel cord, indicating a close, intimate tie.

LiPuma (1988) has described a similar system for the Maring people, who are closely related to the Hageners and live just north of them, in which female blood and male grease (*imbana*) conjoin and bind to produce a fetus. Intrauterine growth occurs as the "mother feeds her baby by passing milk through her umbilical cord. This continues until birth whereupon the midwife . . . severs the cord and the infant starts to feed directly from the breast. . . . Speakers use the term umbilical cord in several contexts to suggest an essential attachment, especially one mediated by women (e.g., a matrilateral kin tie)" (p. 44). This cord is subsequently buried or placed in a hollow of a tree.

The Anganen of the Southern Highlands of Papua New Guinea have a similar ideology of intrauterine growth (Merrett-Balkos 1998):

> The umbilical cord is . . . known as the "road" . . . between mother and child. Vital substance, *ip* [grease], flows from the mother to the unborn child along this path and the cord is the source of life for an infant. The *ip* which flows from mother to child comprises the food a woman eats, but it also conveys aspects of identity to the unborn. (p. 222)

The connection of the fetus to the mother is referred to as *ronga*, "to bind or fasten." *Ronga* and nurturance are sustained after birth through the breast-feeding of milk, and through the use of the netbag (a symbolic extension of the womb that is used as a crib and carrier to transport infants; see MacKenzie 1991; Stewart and Strathern 1997), which has special kinds of leaves placed in it to cushion the child, prevent its spirit from wandering during sleep, and promote its growth (this practice was also used in Hagen and Pangia in the past). The Anganen mothers "consider themselves the archetypical nourishers and growers of children" (Merrett-Balkos, 1998:222) partly because infants consume breast milk that the mother creates from the food that she grows and consumes on the father's land.

As with the Maring, the placenta, *nu*, and its attached umbilical cord are either buried or placed high up in the crook of a tree. The *nu* has to be planted in the clan soil of the child's father, thereby fixing the child to the group of his father while at the same time, through the planting of the umbilical cord, strengthening the tie of the mother's connection to her husband's land. The umbilical cord is known as the "road" and represents relatedness; thus the planting of the cord also affirms the mother's connection to her natal group through the connection that she establishes between affinally related men. Merrett-Balkos states that "'women are like sweet potato runners' and 'women are the road,' or links between groups of men in marriage." This metaphor of women being like sweet potato vines (propagating through connections that spread outward and demonstrating phenomenal abilities to withstand rerooting and replanting) is reflected in the narratives of the Enga people of the Western Highlands Province, who tell how women originally brought the sweet potato into their area, an event that was celebrated by the decoration of bridges over rivers with dangling sweet potato vines and the performance of rituals to celebrate the arrival of this important crop (Wiessner and Tumu 1998; see also O'Hanlon 1989:54 on the idea of "cuttings" as expressive of maternal relationships). Interestingly, there was a taboo on eating sweet potato cooked in ashes during the fertility-seeking Female Spirit cult performances in the Enga, Hagen, Pangia, and Duna areas.

Merrett-Balkos explains further that women nowadays give birth to children in mission health care centers, where they are fed from mission supplies and gardens. Each mother receives a section of her child's umbilical cord after the delivery, and she keeps this with her until she returns home and hides it near her residence. The mothers negotiate this arrangement in order to preserve the essentials of their previous cultural practices (Merrett-Balkos 1998: 221).

The placenta and its associated umbilical cord are considered to be the child's "base place." Anganen ideas appear to closely parallel those of Hagen, as we have expressed them above. Merrett-Balkos (1998) writes that "the significance of the bond . . . between a child and its physiological, uterine source is infused with the meaning of the bond between clan members. . . . Tree or ground burial of the placenta is the action which effects this fusion of meaning" (p. 225). In other words, there is a metathesis or analogy between the child's initial "rootedness" in the mother and its subsequent "rootedness" in its paternal clan territory. The analogy is given force by the metonymic action of taking and re-planting the navel string in the clan ground of the father. But although this reveals a need to transform one kind of connection into another, in fact the tie to the mother and her group is permanent, and the act of building on an internal maternal image in order to create an external "male" identity indicates that these aspects of identity are seen to participate in one another as much as they are in some senses opposed. Merrett-Balkos notes that the term for afterbirth, *nu*, is also the general term for string netbag (as it also is among the Duna). It appears also as an enclitic morph in terms for male collectivities such as *amenu*, "brother sets." Merrett-Balkos contrasts *nu* as a term with *mongol*, "road," suggesting that *nu* has male connotations and *mongol* has female ones (1998:229). This is certainly true; but it is equally interesting that an idiom of male collectivity is founded on an image that is in primordial terms female.

The same can be said of the image found among the Anganen (as well as the Daribi, Foi and Wiru peoples) likening pearl shells to eggs. Pearl shells are one of the categories of male wealth used to secure the reproduction of the clan through payment of bride-prices. Yet in comparing them to eggs, it is clear that men compare their use of male wealth to the production of eggs by female birds. This comparison parallels that of the placenta as a female symbol to the cordyline or banana as a male symbol in the practices noted above. Merrett-Balkos (1998:231) argues that for the Anganen, "womanhood can only be constituted and reflected upon after the mode of being for men." Yet, from another viewpoint, this mode of being for men is also partly modeled on female reproductive processes. Perhaps this point helps to shed light on the phenomenon Merrett-Balkos refers to briefly, the Anganen women's staging of a mass protest at the Catholic mission in 1970. That is, female images are in practice as much a potential source for collective action as are male ones. We might expect this from the general proposition that same-sex idioms relate to the collective, cross-sex ones to individualized realms of action that Merrett-Balkos cites (1998:233); however, cross-sex idioms also are often the basis for collective relationships between groups.

Among the Wiru speakers of Pangia, conception is thought to occur when male and female grease come together and mix, as in Hagen. The growth of girls was said to be faster than that of boys because girls were thought to have a rope leading from their breasts down to their vagina that facilitated their physical development. The placement of this rope also may explain why it was thought to be dangerous to conceive a second child while suckling one, because the semen could enter the mother's milk, pollute it, and kill the child at the breast.

For the Duna, ideas of conception involve the mixing of male "water" and female blood but not grease. This fits with their humoral system, which does not rely on grease as much as the Melpa, Maring, and Anganen ones do, but is based on ideas of blood and water, with water partly taking the place of grease. The Duna also believe that the child grows in utero through the foods that the mother eats, which are thought to replenish/fortify her blood, which then enters the growing fetus through the umbilical cord.

The comparative materials we have assembled here from a range of areas in the Highlands (Hagen, Anganen, Pangia, Duna, Maring) all point clearly to the conclusion that nurturance of the child in utero is thought to take place and that physiological concepts of "ropes" connecting parts of the female body are sometimes brought into play in order to explain how this nurturance takes place. It is consistent with these notions that a pregnant woman is expected to have certain food preferences, because the food she consumes can affect the fetus and its growth. Further, the powerful symbolic actions associated with the placenta and the umbilical cord show that this idea of nurturance is used as a productive metaphor to link "rootedness" and identity. Plants are clearly nurtured by the "grease" in the earth, and children are clearly nurtured by their mothers in the womb and by the food grown on their father's land through the joint efforts of the maternal and paternal sides after the child is weaned.

Procreation and notions of conception and fertility have been of interest to ethnographers working in Papua New Guinea because of their fundamental importance in defining ritual practice and in defining kinship relations (see Jorgensen 1983a for examples). For the Telefolmin of the West Sepik Province of Papua New Guinea, with whom Jorgensen worked, fetal formation was said to be "the combination of male and female sexual fluids in the womb" (1983b:60). Roy Wagner (1983) also describes this joining of substances for the Daribi of Chimbu Province in Papua New Guinea, for whom the human embryo is said to be formed by semen and uterine blood: "The outer layer of the embryo, and the resulting human being, is thus formed by the father, whereas the blood and internal organs are provided by the mother" (p. 76). Interestingly, the source of semen in men is described as flowing through a nexus of ropes called *agwa*—not unlike the female rope system described by the Hagener Ru-Kundil. One further example of the influence of the combination of male and female substance in the formation of the fetus comes from the work of Aletta Biersack among the Paiela of the Enga Province in Papua New Guinea, where "semen, it is thought, must wrap around menstrual blood many times to keep it from 'coming outside' if the woman is to conceive" (1983:85). The image here is the same as that in Hagen. Whatever the particularities of the ideas involved, it is striking that in all cases a combination of substances is seen as necessary for conception.

We will see in chapter 6 a continuation of this theme of conception and fertility through the detailed description of a cult in the Western Highlands Province of Papua New Guinea called Kor Wöp. The Wöp celebrated male fertility power, as well as fertility in general, and it also employed female symbolism, which implied the alliance of the sexes in the work of reproduction. The Wöp spirit was said to make women become pregnant. Thus, the spirit world was also seen as an active agent in fertility.

## REFERENCES

Bernstein, Jay H. 1997. *Spirits Captured in Stone.* London: Lynne Rienner.

Biersack, Aletta. 1983. Bound blood: Paiela "conception" theory interpreted. *Mankind* 14(1):85–100.

Biersack, Aletta (ed.). 1995. *Papuan Borderlands.* Ann Arbor: University of Michigan Press.

Blackwood, Beatrice. 1935. *Both Sides of Buka Passage.* Oxford: Clarendon Press.

Bromley, H. Myron. 1965. The even and the odd: Basic economic concepts of the Grand Valley Dani of Irian Barat. Ms.

Frankel, Stephen. 1986. *The Huli Response to Illness.* Cambridge: Cambridge University Press.

Glick, L. 1963. Foundations of a primitive medical system: The Gimi of the New Guinea Highlands. Ph.D. dissertation, University of Pennsylvania.

Hauser-Schäublin, Brigitta. 1995. Puberty rites, women's naven, and initiation. In N. C. Lutkehaus and P. B. Roscoe, eds., *Gender Rituals: Female Initiation in Melanesia*, pp. 33–53. New York and London: Routledge.

Hayano, D. M. 1974. Misfortune and traditional political leadership among the Tauna Awa of New Guinea. *Oceania* 45(1):18–26.

Jorgensen, Dan. 1983a. Introduction: The facts of life, Papua New Guinea style. *Mankind* 14(1):1–11.

Jorgensen, Dan. 1983b. Mirroring nature? Men's and women's models of conception in Telefolmin. *Mankind* 14(1):57–65.

LiPuma, Edward. 1988. *The Gift of Kinship: Structure and Practice in Maring Social Organization.* Cambridge: Cambridge University Press.

Lutkehaus, Nancy C. 1995. Gender metaphors: Female Rituals as Cultural Models in Manam. In N. C. Lutkehaus and P. B. Roscoe, eds., *Gender Rituals: Female Initiation in Melanesia*, pp. 183–204. New York and London: Routledge.

MacDonald, Mary N. 1991. *Mararoko: A Study in Melanesian Religion.* New York: Peter Lang.

MacKenzie, Maureen. 1991. *Androgynous Objects: String Bags and Gender in Central New Guinea.* Amsterdam: Harwood Academic Publishers.

Meggitt, M. J. 1965. The Mae Enga of Papua New Guinea. In P. Lawrence and M. J. Meggitt, eds., *Gods, Ghosts and Men in Melanesia*, pp. 105–131. Melbourne: Oxford University Press.

Meigs, Anna. 1984. *Food, Sex, and Pollution: A New Guinea Religion.* New Brunswick, NJ: Rutgers University Press.

Merrett-Balkos, Leanne. 1998. Just add water: Remaking women through childbirth, Anganen, Southern Highlands, Papua New Guinea. In Kalpana Ram and Margaret Jolly, eds., *Maternities and Modernities: Colonial and Postcolonial Experiences in Asia and the Pacific*, pp. 213–238. Cambridge: Cambridge University Press.

O'Brien, Denise. 1970. The economics of Dani marriage: An analysis of marriage payments in a highlands New Guinea society. Ph.D. dissertation, Yale University.

O'Hanlon, Michael. 1989. *Reading the Skin: Adornment, Display and Society among the Wahgi*. Bathurst, New South Wales: Crawford House Press.

Riesenfeld, A. 1950. *The Megalithic Culture of Melanesia*. Leiden: E. Brill.

Sillitoe, Paul. 1985. Divide and no-one rules: The implications of sexual divisons of labour in the Papua New Guinea Highlands. *Man* n.s. 20(3):494–522.

Sillitoe, Paul. 1996. *A Place Against Time: Land and Environment in the Papua New Guinea Highlands*. Amsterdam: Harwood Academic Publishers.

Stewart, Pamela. 1998. Ritual trackways and sacred paths of fertility. In Jelle Miedema, Cecilia Ode, and Rien Dam, eds., *Perspectives on the Bird's Head of Irian Jaya, Indonesia: Proceedings of the Conference, Leiden, 13–17 October 1997*, pp. 275–289. Amsterdam and Atlanta: Rodopi.

Stewart, Pamela J., and Andrew Strathern. 1997. Netbags revisited: Cultural narratives from Papua New Guinea. *Pacific Studies.* 20(2):1–30.

Stewart, Pamela J., and Andrew Strathern. 1999a. Female spirit cults as a window on gender relations in the Highlands of Papua New Guinea. *Journal of the Royal Anthropological Institute* 5(3):345–360.

Stewart, Pamela J., and Andrew Strathern. 1999b. Politics and poetics mirrored in indigenous stone objects from Papua New Guinea. *Journal of the Polynesian Society* 108(1):69–90.

Strathern, Andrew, and Pamela J. Stewart. 1998a. Embodiment and communication: Two Frames for the Analysis of Ritual. *Social Anthropology* 6(2):237–251.

Strathern, Andrew, and Pamela J. Stewart. 1998b. Melpa and Nuer ideas of life and death: The rebirth of a comparison. In Michael Lambek and A. J. Strathern, eds., *Bodies and Persons: Comparative Perspectives from Africa and Melanesia*, pp 232–251. Cambridge: Cambridge University Press.

Strathern, Andrew, and Pamela J. Stewart. 2000. *The Python's Back: Pathways of Comparison Between Indonesia and Melanesia*. Westport, CT: Bergin and Garvey.

Wagner, Roy. 1983. The ends of innocence: Conception and seduction among the Daribi of Karimui and the Barok of New Ireland. *Mankind* 14(1):75–83.

Wiessner, Polly, and Akii Tumu. 1998. *Historical Vines*. Washington DC: Smithsonian Institution Press.

Williams, F. E. 1969. *Papuans of the Trans-Fly*. London: Oxford University Press.

# CHAPTER 6

# The Wöp Cult: Water Power

*Pamela J. Stewart and Andrew Strathern*

In this chapter we describe a cult centered on bringing fertility and vitality to local communities. Its focus was on water from a spring and the male spirit embodied in the water. The cult belonged to the Mount Hagen area and was called the Kor Wöp. We will begin by describing the people who participated, and then we will discuss the cult's performative elements. These materials date from 1965, when the cult ritual was still being performed.

In the lower part of the Nebilyer Valley, to the south of Mount Hagen township, squeezed against the tall limestone escarpment that divides it from Tambul and the swampy Tomba plain, there live several small groups linked in tribal alliance pairs whose members tended in the past to coalesce for warfare and rituals. In the mid-1960s these groups were following a mixed program of completing a series of spirit cult performances while at the same time avowedly looking to the local Catholic mission and the Australian colonial administration for their future prospects. These groups, like many of those throughout the Highlands of Papua New Guinea, were caught between an impetus to fulfill their own cultural imperatives and an equally strong inclination to seek the benefits of "modernity": roads, vehicles, schools, health services. It is a dilemma that continues to preoccupy the people of the region today. Their problem was that in order to gain the new benefits they desired, they were being asked to give up some of those cultural practices in which their aspirations and wishes for their well-being were embedded.

The area where these concerns were being played out, in terms of spirit cults on the one hand and church and administration work on the other, is known to the people as Kulir. It is the same place which Francesca Merlan and Alan Rumsey in their comprehensive sociolinguistic study called Ku Waru (Merlan and Rumsey 1991:22). Ku Waru means "[at] the edge of the stone," a reference to the limestone wall at the back of the area. In mid-1965 Kulir was used as a term for a putatively distinctive dialect spoken in the area, in contrast with the Meam dialect prevalent in the broader expanses of the Nebilyer Valley to the north. In general, to the Melpa speakers who live still further to the north, around Mount Hagen township, the language of the Nebilyer Valley speakers is known as Temboka. The Kulir version of this language is closer to that spoken in Tambul than that in Meam; this is not by chance, because the Kulir groups have multiple historical connections with Tambul and Tomba. Most particularly the spirit cult rituals they were planning to perform, or had already performed, in mid-1965 were largely ones imported from Tambul, which was seen as an important source of cult power (Didi 1982a, 1982b). Boyope Didi has suggested that one motivation impelling the Tambul groups to develop and export these cults was the poor quality of the Tambul soil and the cold, high-altitude climate there. By holding these fertility cult rituals they hoped to improve the fertility of their soil, and by exporting them they acquired much-needed wealth items that could be used for bride-price and other exchange payments (Didi 1982a, 1982b; Strathern and Stewart n.d.).

This suggestion is plausible, and it points to the fact that cults and their movements in space belong to ecological and historical contexts (see Sillitoe 1996; Strathern and Stewart 1998; Wiessner and Tumu 1998). The investigations in the Kulir area in 1965 revealed that the selective appropriation of cults was used as a means of internal differentiation of identities among the small and historically hard-pressed Kulir groups. Each group tended to have taken up one of a range of available cult "options," and the choices they made both reflected and influenced perceptions of ties with other groups in the vicinity, including the Tambul groups.

The Kulir groups all lived close to the dividing limestone wall. They had nowhere to expand, and their numbers in the past had been reduced in warfare, to the extent that their alliance pairs at the level of the tribe were equivalent in population sizes to the alliances of small clans within tribes among stronger neighboring groups such as the Ulka, Kulka, and Ndika to the north. These were groups, then, that must have had a strong awareness of their own historically contingent and marginal situation. Reduced both in numbers and in territory size, they aimed through their cults to boost their continuity and the fertility of their land, to keep their separate existence, and to compete with each other for some special access to ritual power.

The ritual experts who were brought in from the nearby Tambul area to perform for them entered into this competitive context and had to deal with it. In particular, the groups and subgroups that were combining for the cult rituals comprised an alliance pair that had been divided by disputes on other occasions. Bringing them together for the performance was a way of making them share the sacred power of the cult in the form of the spring water that is one of the manifestations of the spirit. It is not very clear how the memory of this significant ritual event was later constructed. Merlan and Rumsey, in their very detailed representation of relations between groups (*talapi*) in Kulir, and in particular of speeches given on political occasions involving the same sets of people we are discussing here, do not appear to have recorded any reference to this sharing of cult activities that had taken place in 1965. Their own initial fieldwork was carried out between 1981 and 1983, almost twenty years after the cult performances recorded here. They frequently write about intergroup relations, seeing these as being in states of historical and experiential flux rather than in terms of a contrast between structure and agency (Merlan and Rumsey 1991:136). Although this is an interesting way to obviate a contrast that has proved problematic in social analyses, partly by regarding the actions of individual actors as socially created (Merlan and Rumsey 1991:136), and therefore on a par with "segmentary identities," it has one drawback: it makes it more difficult to discuss historical continuities.

Yet, the named social categories to which the people whom Merlan and Rumsey studied in 1982–1983 referred as constituting their affirmative social world are clearly labeled with the same names as in 1965. This helps us to bridge the gap in time, and look for continuities and changes. Thus, we may reasonably identify an arena of structure, signaling a certain domain of continuity. Such continuity is of course in practice not a transcendent entity; rather, it is the sediment of the historical work of agency of particular social actors and groups. In turn, however, it becomes the life world that these actors inhabit. Everything in this life world is created, but not all at the same time. Individual, socially created acts of agency feed into one another and into this continuing world of collective social life, whose longer-lasting features can be seen as its "structure."

With this point in mind, it is helpful to note that the kinds of social relations recorded in 1965 between the Kulir groups are clearly reflected in Merlan and Rumsey's detailed delineations from 1982–1983, for example the ongoing enmities between the Epokla–Elya alliance pair and the Koepiya–Kumbuka alliance pair (Epola-Alya and Kopia-Kubuka in Merlan and Rumsey's phonemic transcription). The materials from September 1965 that we present here also show the classic situation of a partial split between the Epokla and the Elya. The Elya were the main cult sponsors, and at times the Epokla had to be persuaded to cooperate. The ritual leaders, whose commands were given to both groups, enjoining their collaboration as a condition of the ritual's success, played an important part in ensuring this circumstantial solidarity and thus in securing payments from both sides for their services. The Epokla and Elya were said in 1965 to have a single place of origin (*möi peng*, "ground head" or origin), and formed a single exogamous community. However, when one of the ritual cult houses was built, it was said that there had been some contention between the two groups and they had almost fought. The chief ritual expert for the performance reminded them of this later, when the Elya wanted to complete a sequence of cult activity without the Epokla. He told them:

> You are all of one ancestral father. He was a polygynist who married different wives, and now you have different men's houses as descendants of these wives and you live in different places, but you are still "men of one penis" [*wuö noimb tenda*]. The bones [cult stones] of the Kor Wöp [Male Spirit] also have been buried together in this place, some given by Epokla and some by Elya.

If the two sides were to split apart or fail to combine for the cult, the expert added, this would be a denial of their ultimate ancestral co-identity, which would cause them to lose the "grease" in their penises (*wuö noimb nu moklmba*, "in the men's penises there will be water"), and would result in the "spilling out" of the cult stones (*kor ku oi nimba*) from their proper resting places. This would be equivalent to their willful self-destruction, because their shared totemic emblem, the *mi*, would then "eat" (i.e., kill) them, according to an explanation given by one field assistant.

Through such references to the cult's essential purpose of fertility, conjoined with the imperative of solidarity, the ritual expert insisted on keeping the combined performance on track. In this way the ongoing historical competition over access to ritual powers, between the Epokla-Elya alliance pair and other such paired groups, was maintained.

These same considerations strongly influenced the response of the Kulir groups in the 1960s to the presence of the new forces of administration and the Catholic Church. In this new context they were peripheral. Their leaders, engaged in organizing the spirit cults, were at the same time trying to discover how best to attract government resources to their area and how to accommodate the wishes of the Catholic missionaries. The cult areas that were surveyed were all located at the back of the new mission station, which was built on the site of a ceremonial dancing ground. Cult leaders were quick to declare that in response to the mission's wishes, they had already given up much of their practice of ancestor worship and were no longer concerned as much with sorcery, because they were "afraid of the Catholic Father and of God." They were anxious to secure the building of a government road into the new station area and to have prospects of doing contract labor on a large new highway that was projected to run from Mount Hagen township to the Southern Highlands towns of Ialibu and Mendi. They declared that they were already partly "men of law," who just wanted to get these spirit cults over and done with. The next generation, who would have been initiated into the next cycle of performances, would fully convert to the ways of the mission and the colonial government.

Why, then, did they hold the cult performances? Quite clearly, these cults represented a long-term investment to obtain fertility and continuity that did not need to be repeated until another generation had grown to sexual maturity, a period of some twenty years. With their indigenous imported spirit powers on their side, they could tackle getting the best out of the new rituals brought to them by the white outsiders: rituals whose meanings and social requirements they only partially grasped.

As we have noted, in 1965 the Elya group was sponsoring a performance of the Wöp cult ritual. This cult has as its central image of power the notion of a spring of water bubbling up spontaneously from the ground and forming a stream. The spot where such a spring is found becomes incorporated into the cult center, and the first step taken to institute the cult is to call in a ritual expert from the Tambul/Tomba area to "manage" the spring. The ritual expert clears the area round the spring, defines where cult fences should be built, and makes a place for the spring to flow downward from its head (*peng*) to a lower outlet (its *por*, or back) in an unimpeded channel. The spring is called the "eye of the spirit" (*kor mong* or *kor kik mong*, "the spirit's ashes' eye"). There may be two springs, one called "the open one" and the other "the closed one" (*kumbeli mökeli rakl*). The adult men who participate in the cult drink spring water offered them by the expert, who also tests the water and drinks from it to help his body feel good (*pral*).

The ritual expert who officiated at the Elya performance, Raklpa, said that when he drank the water, his *muntmong pral nimba wangndorom* (his heart felt refreshed and at ease). He emphasized the good effects on his body by placing his hands on his chest and wiping them over his skin constantly as he spoke. The water was explicitly said to assist the men's wives to bear sons, who were needed to replace males killed in warfare. The gushing of the spring water is thus clearly thought of as an image of fertility power, and the water contributes to the fluids that pass between the sexes in intercourse, inducing enhanced fertility. The surrounds of the spring are adorned with decorative ferns (*nöng*). The Wöp is a cult of water power, and water is seen equally as a source of human fertility and fertility of the ground. The sacred spring water contributes to human "humors" in this sense, increasing their vitality and potency. When the men wish to drink the spring water, they send a pair of young boys, neophytes in the cult, to fetch it for them.

A general conspectus of the Wöp cult practices was given by a leader of one of the groups neighboring the Epokla-Elya, the Rokla-Wanika. The leader was of the Wanika group in this alliance pair. The following is a transcript of his explanatory speech:

We learn the custom from others—the Köwul men of Tambul come and make rituals and spells [*mön*] for us. Then a big man is sick or pigs grow slowly, and we say it is the Kor Wöp who does this. If our skin is poor, we send talk to the big man and tell him we are sick because of Kor Wöp. We get the ritual expert [*mön wuö*] in, and he tells us that a ritual performance [*kor mön*] is required, and we should cut bananas and get pigs. He shows us the place of Kor Wöp, and we cut the bush and put a stake [*kor porembil*] as a marker in the place. We cook pigs there, and the *mön wuö* finds stones that make men sick. Pig's blood is put on the stones, and they are hidden in one place. Such a stone may have a leg, nose, eye, or finger. . . . These are the spirit's bones [*kor ombil*]. Some of the stones are long, and some are round with a hole—they are male and female. We kill pigs when we set up the *kor porembil.* Then we build a tall house, without walls and a covered roof at the top only. It has a high central post—they use the bark of the tree *nde köngon* for the roof. This is the tower house [*manga tamand*]. Another is the cooking house [*röng el manga*]—if they sleep on the site or they find a piece of pork to cook, they go there. If we take pork or live pigs in, we taboo the meat to the women. We cook pigs there. We won't cut pieces of pork for our sisters, or they would bear male children that would be with their fathers [i.e., increase male offspring outside of the group because these sisters marry exogamously]. We give this meat to our wives so that they will bear their own children for us. Our wives eat the pork, and if they become pregnant, it is the Kor Wöp who makes this to be, although God does this for some of the women.

When we have cooked these pigs, we look at our living pigs, and when they are big, we say now we are ready to cook the Wöp proper. Some men have pigs and others do not, and we give a *kibung* to them [advise them in a meeting] and then they prepare their pigs. We watch the progress of the pigs, and when they are ready, the participants must get some marsupials. They mark the day about three or four years ahead. Men who can hunt find marsupials. If not, we pay pearl shells and axes to another group for marsupials they have caught. We send talk to our maternal kin, cross-cousins or brothers-in-law, to do this, and so we give them pay for their hard work with money, axes, and pearl shells.

We make a huge fence round the Wöp enclosure. Our in-laws and cross-cousins bring decorations and bamboo tubes of Campnosperma tree oil [*kopong nde*] to us inside the cult fence. The fence is a prohibition on people to come inside, like a lock on a door. The men decorate themselves: face paint, shells on the neck, and the like. They dance inside the enclosure. Others come to look. The men break out of the fence and make a good dance. We put on the bark belt, the baler shell on the forehead [*ndum*], *köi ketepa* [long headdresses of the King of Saxony bird], and face paint, and others all admire these when they see us. Spectators say this clan has made a good dance, and will not die quickly; they will live to be old, only later they will die; their skin is big.

Men without pigs cook marsupials, and these are eaten. They look at us, and it is finished. We kill pigs and pay those who brought us decorations with pork.

A *mön wuö* comes and works *mön* [makes spells] for us, and we pay him with baler shells, money, pearl shells, axes, pigs. Otherwise the *mön wuö* would talk badly of us when he went back to his own place. The head and backbones and legs of pig are given, and the *mön wuö* takes it all. . . .

Other men will not tell you another story, this one only. I have seen the Wöp myself and know about it.

There are many large groups, Ndika and Mokei, all over the mountain, but only one man knows the source [*pukl*] of the spells [*kor mön*] for the Wöp. We note that his talk is straight and men's skin is good and pigs grow fat and so we give him pay. It is the Köwul Mundke group who are the source of this ritual power and of the Wöp—they live at Tambul. There are Okopuke experts [from the northeast of the Nebilyer Valley, toward Hagen] for the Wöp also now.

The pigs are not enough by themselves—the marsupials must also be cooked for it [the ritual] to go straight—not birds, but all kinds of marsupials.

The pigs and marsupials are cooked in separate earth ovens. The marsupial meat is not given to the women to eat, but the pork is.

A man is small when he does not cook the *kor*, but big when he does.

Several points in this summary narrative are notable. In sequence, the elements the leader emphasized are the following:

1. The cult knowledge comes from Tambul and is exercised by a ritual expert belonging to the Mundke tribe.
2. The need to institute the cult ritual comes from the sickness of leaders and poor quality of the pig herds.
3. They call into the area an expert who "shows us the place of Kor Wöp." This is the water spring, which the leader never mentions by name in his narrative. This apparent "omission" probably reflects a reluctance by the leader to show the spring site to outsiders, and therefore indicates the importance of the spring to the cult's inner meaning and purpose.
4. The ritual expert finds the cult stones of the Wöp. Most, though not all, of the regional spirit cults had these stones as repositories of the spirit's power, and pigs were sacrificed at the ritual stake set up as the spirit's marker, the *porembil*, to anoint the stones with their blood. The cult therefore establishes a range of ritual foci at which substance transfers take place. For the Wöp there is a double focus on the cult stones and the spring water. The *porembil* stake also acts as a taboo sign, or *mi*, to ward off sickness sent by the Wöp spirit, and the sacrifices at it are made with this purpose in mind.
5. Under the directions of the expert, the men build the cult houses and fences separating them. The two main houses described are the *klöng ekl nggu*, the "food roasting house," and the *manga tamand*, the "central post house" or tall tower house. The main significance of these houses was that the participants cooked different parts of pigs or marsupials in them at different times. All of the cults had quite specific rules separating the places where certain foods could be cooked and distributed for consumption. It is not easy to determine the exact rationale for all these divisions, but three elements stand out: the separation of ovens used for cooking sweet potatoes from those for pork; the separation of ovens for pork and those for marsupial meat; and the separation of sacrifices in the food roasting house and those in the tower house—only in the latter were pigs' livers cooked and later cut up in stone mortars (*kung kaemb ku*) for distribution to participants.
6. The leader stresses that this cult ritual is for in-group purposes. Sacrificial meat is not given to sisters who have married elsewhere, because this would benefit the agnatic continuity and strength of other groups. The competitive element shows clearly here. The Wöp cult quite specifically aimed at enhancing the fertility of its male participants' wives, and although the leader does not explicitly say so, the expert took parts of the pigs' livers, strongly associated with male power/strength, and gave these to women. Women decorated themselves elaborately and joined in the final dance celebration. Neither of these two features is found in the Amb Kor, the Female Spirit cult (Strathern and Stewart 1998, 2000).
7. The cult ritual performance ends with a massive dance display, called *kor poke*, a name that is particular to this cult context. The dance combines the styles of two other ceremonial dances, known as *mör* and *kanan*.
8. It is important to hire an effective expert and to pay him handsomely; otherwise the cult sponsors would be criticized and would lose the prestige they hope to gain.

9. Marsupials must be cooked in addition to pork. The marsupial meat is not shared with the women. This element seems to relate strongly to the cult's origin place in Tambul, a high-altitude forested area where marsupials are plentiful. The Kulir men sometimes had to ask their extraclan relatives to help them hunt for marsupials to use. Their own young men might hunt them and keep them alive for a while before presenting them to the older men in return for a reward of special foods, such as taro and banana. Possibly these practices reflect a time when there was a differently gendered dynamic to the practices in the cult, later modified when there was a greater reliance on pigs, sweet potatoes, and female labor (compare Wiessner and Tumu 1998). It is possible that marsupial meat was thought to stimulate male virility and therefore would be inappropriate to share with females.
10. The results of the *kor* show in people's *bodies* and abilities or mind: "A man is small when he does not perform the Wöp, big when he does." Here "small" means both physically small and socially insignificant, and "big" means both healthy and important.

Elements in the Wöp that distinguish it from the Amb Kor performances (discussed in Chapter 5) are the "eye of the spirit," the spring; the distribution of pieces of liver to women inside the enclosure; the participation of women in the final dance; the apparent lack of traditions of finding the cult stones through dreams; and the separate cooking of marsupials, for male consumption only. In other respects these two cults and the others that had proliferated in the Kulir area can be seen as variations on a set of common themes. For example, there is a basic triadic division of the cult area, with a guest house in the first part, a sacrifice house in the second, and a most significant sacrificial area in the third. The "food-roasting house" of the Wöp is clearly like the "*möri* leaf house" of the Amb Kor. In both there is a rigid division of the performers into the "men's house" and "women's house" sides, which have their separate seating in the sacrificial house. Also, in both the cult stones are seen as having agency: they reveal themselves to the founders, and they do so when the Spirit has made someone sick. The stones, described as the bones of the spirit, also are of various shapes, elongated and round, and although the Wöp spirit is male, some of its stones were said to be female, emphasizing the sexual metaphor of fertility that underlies the cult practices and the recognition of male and female aspects within a single sex. The Mundke (Mundika) expert who officiated for the Epokla-Elya, Kaemb, said that the two main types of Wöp stones were called Tambul Kela Kömök ("red ocher leader from Tambul") and Tambul Keke, one a mortar and the other a pestle, described as "pig liver stone" and "pig-killing-stick stone," respectively. An element that is foregrounded in one cult may be present but muted in the other. The spring water is central to the Wöp, but in the Amb Kor, also the experts offer bespelled water to the participants, telling them that this will make their stomachs clean and healthy, whereas in the Wöp they drink the water in order to make themselves able to transmit male fertility.

The special importance of water to the Wöp is not something that has to be deduced or inferred analytically. It is a part of the shared, conscious model used by participants themselves. The cult leader among the Rokla-Wanika in Kulir explained further:

It is the Kor Wöp that makes our women pregnant and our pigs pregnant and our skins good, our gardens grow well. We take our pigs or our yams and other good vegetables and cook these for Kor Wöp. Our wives will bear male children only if we cook pigs for the Wöp—Wöp gives them the children. [This was affirmed by the ritual experts for the Elya performance also.]

The performers' hair is teased out, and this done by an expert for one shilling or two shillings. . . . When this is done, the hair is not cut afterward, although they say when it is finished, they cut down the cult houses and walk about normally. We don't see the Kor Wöp, who is in the water, but the spirit has come to live in the place and is shown by his stones [*oimbukl*]. The liver of the pig is taken, and this is distributed by the *mön wuö* to the wives of the group, and these bear male children and they feed pigs successfully.

When the *mön wuö* talks, we are very quiet. The *mön wuö* holds the pig's liver, and we sit down . . . and he distributes it to us. If a man talks, he will die. Ten or twenty Mundke *mön wuö* will come and sit down in the middle of us and make their *mön* to us. We pay them with pigs, pearl shells, balers, axes, and money.

The *kor mön wuö* do not go down to the spring [*kor mong*]. This is water for drinking only. It is at the other houses that the *mön* is performed.

If a man sleeps at the head of the river and is sick, it is Kor Wöp who kills him. The water spurts up by itself, it jumps and jumps, and the men drink from it. Men dig down and find the spring coming up.

We find new pearl shells, new cordyline rear coverings, new bark belts and head dresses [ *kera klapa*]. The water fills up a long bamboo, and it helps the men to have a fat, strong skin when they perform their dance. We drink the *kor mong* [the spring water] and our dances are good.

Notable in this account is the quite explicit reference to the idea that the Wöp gives male children to the wives of the men who make the sacrifices to it. These sons, much needed in times of warfare, are given in return for the gift of the sacrifices. Further, the consecrated pig's liver cooked under the tower house also carries the power to confer male children, and is fed directly to the wives for this purpose. Once again the speaker downplays the significance of the spring water, saying that the experts do not perform rituals at it; "it is just drinking water." The opposite is true, because culminating rituals in the cult include the casting into the spring of sugarcane fragments and expensive Campnosperma tree oil (*kopong keta kae*, "grease face good"), followed by the closing of the "spirit eye," sealing its powers in the ground and controlling its potentially dangerous aspects. Trees and bushes are felled over the site, obscuring and protecting it. The Campnosperma tree oil is used for decorating the body. It is red, symbolizing fertility, blood, and well-being. Among some Highland peoples, such as the Foi, this tree and its oil have an association with menstrual blood (see Weiner 1995:159ff.), and therefore with fertility.

The water of the spirit is potent as an external topical application as well as an internal medicine. One man explained, "The stones of Kor Wöp [those used in the cult] are connected with procreation, and the *kor mong* [spring water] with the custom whereby women who are pregnant as a result of mixing their grease with that of their men regularly go down to the water to wash their belly. It is this water that makes the child's body grow straight, forms its hands and feet; hence this is the secret of Kor Wöp." (This man also declared that the Wöp cult stones had true power, whereas those for the Amb Kor (Female Spirit) cult were just river stones.)

During the Wöp cult ritual, experts killed pigs and chanted a spell over them before they were taken to be cooked in the final ceremony. During the spell the expert closed the eyes and ears of the pigs with mountain moss steeped in pig's blood, calling on everything to "stick" (*römb*), that is, to stay fertile, to make grease (*kopong*) (the word for grease is the same as for semen and breast milk). The cult's theme of fertility was pursued further in the construction of a "magic garden" (Strauss and Tischner 1962:419)—a metaphor for the pregnant body and a representation of horticultural sustainability. At a later point in the ritual sequence, the cult participants encircled the magic garden. All the men held onto a long, thick *keunga* vine, decorated with *nöng* ferns and bespelled by the experts. They then descended upon the garden and tore away pieces of it that would later be pushed down into the "eye" of the Spirit's spring. The men performed the vine dance to enhance their longevity and the solidarity of their groups. This ritual sequence was called *peng mumuk*, "holding the head together." Cult stones were buried in the local earth after being liberally anointed with pig's blood and oil, and wrapped in moss and ferns to keep them "cool." This was done to bring the ground long-term fertility and to keep it from becoming "dry" (i.e., without grease/vitality).

Other ritual sequences for the cult also involved the presentation of substances to the earth, predominantly pig's blood and Campnosperma oil. In one sequence prior to the final dance, for example, the celebrants were required to bring in two tall saplings of the *yamkamb* tree which were then set into prepared holes on either side of the entrance-way into the cult area just in front of the main woven fence that separated this area from the nearby ceremonial ground used for the public dance at the cult's climax. The chief ritual expert, Raklpa, and his associates scraped the bark off the lower part of these posts in order to make their "skin" good and smooth. This ritual act was a sign (*to*) that people's skins should be good and they should be free from sickness. Then, with a mass of forest moss, the chief ritual expert applied Campnosperma oil to the post, then pig's blood, and finally rubbed it with charcoal (*ndip öruma*) which had been prepared earlier in the tower house. He attached a piece of tough pandanus leaf and *nöng* ferns to the lower end of each post and then added the nuts of a particular tree and the nest of a hornet (*pilima*), along with a small live river fish (*oma tilik*). These were all adjunct items (*tamb-mel*) to assist in the project of fertility. The expert and his associates bound the posts round with *kan towakl*, the same kind of tough creeper rope that was used in the *peng mumuk* sequence. The celebrants held the posts up and the posts were allowed to descend quietly into the holes dug for them on either side of the entry way to the cult area; the spectators were expected to remain silent. (The quiet periods are to ensure that the spirit is not annoyed or frightened by noises.) Not only did the spectators have to stay quiet while the posts were brought out from the enclosure, but they were told to listen for shouting from any other direction. If there was any, this would mean that a person from that area would die. At the end of the cult ritual, the enclosure fence was violently cut down, but there was a strict taboo on disturbing the posts, again on penalty of expected death. Considerable solemnity therefore surrounded this gift to the earth.

The surface of the posts was treated like the skin on a human body, and the chief expert explicitly said that this was intended to make people's skins good (*köng ama ru tepa moklangka*). Each *tamb-mel* used had an explanation attached to it. The hornet's nest was said to be used by the insect to attach itself to trees and remain firm there, so the crops would remain firm in the fields. The fish was slippery, and in the same way sickness would slip from people's skins and they would be well. The nut, *kuklumb kekrakl*, is found high in the tree and is enclosed by a strong shell resistant to boring insects. Raklpa added; *elim-nga king eng nomba kae etem, wamb ama noman ngoromen* (its skin is shiny and good, people really like it); hence it, too, is a mark that people's skins will be good and they will live long.

All of these examples clearly show the cosmic participatory logic at the heart of these ritual actions. The concern is with the human body. Elements of the environment are brought into play in the pursuit of health for the body. Humans are thus assimilated to the outer world, especially the world of the forest, and at the same time they selectively employ it for their own ends.

These acts of assertive agency were accompanied by ones celebrating the life of the group. Immediately after completing the complex technical job of assembling the right elements for the tree-planting ritual, Raklpa led the celebrants back into the enclosure to the cooking house, where he distributed a single sweet potato to each man and told them to eat these with their heads down, silently and in unison, all of them finishing their meal at the same time. Anyone out of step with this sequence might cause a danger of death in the group. One man did finish early—a chief rival of the Elya cult sponsor, a "boss boy" (a term used by the colonial powers to designate a particular man who had a set of administrative duties in a certain area) among the paired Epokla group. His action may have been deliberate.

The overall ritual, then, like many others found cross-culturally, dramatically expressed and condensed human aims and action patterns in a speeded-up form: from a specialized ritual act by an individual expert the action moved swiftly to a solemn act of solidarity (and an individual transgression of this), all tied in with the aim of harnessing the cosmos to human ends while harmonizing humans with one another. This group solidarity also extended to the women in the community, who observed various taboos and restrictions along with those that the men observed (Stewart and Strathern 1999). Raklpa, well aware of the new presence of the Catholic Church in the area, constantly commented that all this was good and virtuous, the ritual had no harmful intentions in it, and though he practiced his own art in a sincere way, he had sent his son to the Catholic school to learn the secrets of the new *mön* (ritual knowledge) taught there. When, at the end of the performance, it was announced that a man among the Okopuke group some miles away, former enemies of the Kulir groups, had died, putatively of "poison," just before the Elya leaders announced that they would hold their final dance, Raklpa insisted that he knew no reason for the coincidence and had nothing to do with it. His own work was for the good of everyone. Others thought that there might be some connection between the events, suggesting that the dance had been delayed by the local leaders as a ploy until the man died, and that holding it amounted to a celebration of the death. This was never corroborated. In its form, however, it reminds us of the rivalrous political context into which cosmic acts of sacrifice could be placed, although for the cult experts, and perhaps the bulk of the community, these frames were kept separate: the cult's aims were positive, no matter what other factors affected the timing of its various stages.

The water of the spring in the Wöp cult is specific evidence of the life-giving power of the earth, here imaged as a male spirit able to facilitate women's powers of reproduction and their capacity to bear male children through sexual intercourse. The idea of the Wöp spirit joins together a sense of the cosmos and a sense of personal agency. The spring is not just water, it is the channel for the spirit's agency. And equally, putting on the cult ritual as a complex performance and as a means of establishing the name of its sponsors—in the case discussed, the Elya in conjunction with their allies the Epokla—is an expression both of dependence on the imagined world of the cosmos and on the enacted world of personal leadership, commitment, and participation by both sexes in the overall enterprise. The preparations for the cult ritual took many years and were set deeply into the nexus of historical animosities, rivalries, and alliances that characterized this marginal part of the Nebilyer Valley. The Elya cult leader, for example, saw the cult both as a way of asserting his and his group's preeminence within the alliance pair of Epokla-Elya and as a means of attracting supporters for himself in an upcoming local government council election in which the Elya and the Epokla were to be combined in one constituency. Such ambitions, however, are cycled through a cosmic field of wider relationships within which political and economic ends are seen as part and parcel of a religious worldview and its values, values that encompass both sexes in an enduring sense of their place within the environment on which they depend for the reproduction of life. The flow of humors and substances is seen as providing the dynamic means for the cosmos to be maintained and, within that, for the fortunes and desires of individuals to be realized.

As noted earlier in this chapter, the Nebilyer people were also faced with historical dilemmas and conflicting demands on their energies placed on them by government and missionary representatives. The government wanted their labor for road work, and the Catholic mission was bent on replacing their old sense of the cosmos with a new one centered on a Christian God, to which the people responded with a mixture of opportunism, struggles to understand, and pragmatic efforts to accommodate the old and the new together. On the one hand, they declared that they had given up the practice of building sacrificial huts for the skulls of deceased group members. On the other hand, each group in the Kulir area had a site for one or another of the spirit cults that came from the Tambul area, and either had held a ritual or was planning one in the near future. Concerned to gather both their past and their future into the complexities of their present life, they held on to certain symbols as experiential markers of real powers that could not be ignored. Along with the government's command of the police and the missionaries' words about the power of God, the image of the spring water of the Wöp stood for them as a sign of their own locally realized, cosmically placed agency.

The emphasis on fluids in cult practices such as the Wöp was an expression of how the people saw their own bodily fluids in a dynamic relationship with the fluids of the wider environment within which they lived. Ritual experts who served as healers outside of cult contexts often invoked the powers of water to dispel sickness from the human body. One spell collected in 1964 from the ritual expert Moka among the Hagen people sent "bad blood," which was causing a sickness for a man, away through the watercourses that flowed from the expert's high mountain location downward to the west and northwest, and out to the great junction of rivers between the Highlands and the Sepik region guarded by two spirit women. In similar spells the junction of the rivers Ndimi and Klai (Jimi and Lai) is mentioned as the place where the two spirit women stand:

Down to the Mökö River,
Down to the banks of the Eimbö River,
Down to the junction with the Aninga River,
Down to the junction with the Ruruk River,
Down to the junction with the Ikik River,
Down to the junction with the Kuni River,
Down to the junction with the Pöyö River,
Down to the junction with the Wakl River,
Down to the junction with the Oktökin River,
There where the two spirit women
    Mak and Piltik stand,
There where the two spirit women
    Pakop and Makop stand.
Where the cassowary stands on one leg,
    I send it down there,
The cassowary kicks it, and
It tumbles away, it closes up, and
There it stays.

This spell gives us a vivid impression of the ritual expert's sense of his own emplacement within a landscape of river waters, whose powers he summoned into himself for his healing activities. It also testifies to the powers of image-making in the expert's own mind and his command of a mental map going well beyond any landscape he had personally experienced. In other words, the spell reflects both the picture of a cosmos and the imprint of the expert's own agency. The intimate connection between the body, the world, and agency here encapsulated is akin to the topic of Chapter 7, also centered on the Hagen area, which we call "Mind Substance."

## REFERENCES


Didi, Boyope K. 1982a. Kuru Kopiaka, Goddess cult in the lower Kaugel Valley of the Tambul Sub-District, Western Highlands Province. *Oral History* 10(1):5–43.

Didi, Boyope K. 1982b. An overview of the traditional cults in the lower Kaugel Valley of the Tambul Sub-District, Western Highlands Province. *Oral History* 10(1):44–87.

Merlan, Fancesca, and Alan Rumsey. 1991. *Ku Waru: Language and Segmentary Politics in the Western Nebilyer Valley, Papua New Guinea.* Cambridge: Cambridge University Press.

Sillitoe, Paul. 1996. *A Place Against Time: Land and Environment in the Papua New Guinea Highlands.* Amsterdam: Harwood Academic Publishers.

Stewart, Pamela J., and Andrew Strathern. 1999. Female spirit cults as a window on gender relations in the highlands of Papua New Guinea. *Journal of the Royal Anthropological Institute* 5(3):345–360.

Strathern, Andrew, and Pamela J. Stewart. 1998. Embodiment and communication: Two frames for the analysis of ritual. *Social Anthropology* 6(2):237–251.

Strathern, Andrew, and Pamela J. Stewart. 2000. *The Python's Back: Pathways of Comparison Between Indonesia and Melanesia.* Westport, CT: Bergin and Garvey.

Strathern, Andrew, and Pamela J. Stewart n.d. Cults, closures, and collaborations. For a volume containing a collection of papers from the "Women in Male Rituals of New Guinea" session, convened by Pascale Bonnemère, at the 1999 Association for Social Anthropology in Oceania meeting, Hilo, Hawaii.

Strauss, Hermann, and Herbert Tischner. 1962. *Die Mi-Kultur der Hagenberg Stämme.* Hamburg: Cram, de Gruyter.

Weiner, James. 1995. *The Lost Drum: The Myth of Sexuality in Papua New Guinea and Beyond.* Madison: University of Wisconsin Press.

Wiessner, Polly, and Akii Tumu. 1998. *Historical Vines.* Washington DC: Smithsonian Institution Press.

# CHAPTER 7

# Mind Substance

*Pamela J. Stewart and Andrew Strathern*

In this chapter we discuss what we call "mind substance," that which is processed by both the conscious and the unconscious mind and is shared, to one extent or another, outward through relationships with other people, objects, and the environment. The materials that we present are based on an indigenous Hagen notion of ***noman***, which has been discussed as mind or will (A. Strathern 1981; M. Strathern 1988; Stewart and Strathern 2000; Strathern and Stewart 1998, 1999b). Here we develop, through the use of specialized interview materials, the concept of the ***noman*** as emblematic of conscious mind, encompassing the phenomenological stimuli that shape the ***noman*** through experience or "being."

Antonio Damasio writes that

> Consciousness is, in effect, the key to life examined, for better and for worse, our beginner's permit into knowing all about the hunger, the thirst, the sex, the tears, the laughter, the kicks, the punches, the flow of images we call thought, the feelings, the words, the stories, the beliefs, the music and the poetry, the happiness and the ecstasy. At its simplest and most basic level consciousness lets us recognize an irresistible urge to stay above and develop a concern for the self. At its most complex and elaborate level, consciousness helps us develop a concern for other selves and improve the art of life. (1999:5)

Clearly, aspects of what we call the unconscious form and shape the ***noman*** as well. We see through the description of ***noman*** both the transpersonal and the contemplative aspects of the self that we have previously termed the "relational-individual" (Stewart and Strathern 2000). Also, it is clear from these materials that the experiential development of *noman* occurs via flows of mind substance (see in particular the commentary on extract 5 of the texts from Wömndi below).

Spatial imagery predominates in discussions about the *noman*, even though it is said not to be visible in the body as a separate organ. It is *experienced* as being in the cavity of the chest near the heart and the windpipe, the pathway of breath and speech. It has "upper" and "lower" aspects, either of which can prevail over the other and either of which can be multiple or singular. The imagery of upper and lower parts to some extent correlates with a conscious/unconscious distinction, but is better represented as a notion of that which is immediately accessible versus that which is submerged.

Ideas about the interaction of the *noman* or mind with other aspects of the person, including bodily aspects, are of great and enduring significance in Hagen. This does not mean that such ideas are unchanging. Far from it. We have gradually recognized, in looking over field notes from the 1960s and comparing them with materials from the 1990s in Hagen, how ideas have altered over time. Furthermore, we are not dealing here with fixed forms of ideology, but with fluid and sometimes variable notions, as often happens when people try to work out their own models of fundamental realities, basing these models both on experience and on interpretations of experience.

Some detailed discussions centering on the *noman* were held in April 1979 with two men, Wömndi and Ongka. Wömndi was a married man with young children. Ongka was a senior leader (see Strathern and Stewart 1999a, 2000). Both belong to the Kawelka group, and at the time they were living in their respective clan areas at Mbukl and Ngolke in the Dei Council area north of Hagen township.

We present considerable portions of these interviews. Our major purpose is not to extract a single, completely consistent worldview supposedly shared by all Hageners, but rather to show how these two men constructed their own views out of a substratum of notions that certainly held wide currency among Hageners. Their observations indicate how they saw the interaction of what we call mind and body, and how they saw that interaction growing and changing over the life span of the person; how they constructed gender categories; and how they reflected on certain notions that since the 1950s had been introduced along with Christianity in their area. The interviews are snapshots of ideas at a particular time, expressing both continuity and change in historical experience, and reflection on it.

The questions posed also came out of fieldwork in the Hagen area and the information it had brought with it over the years since 1964. Thus these interviews were a means of testing and exploring the knowledge that had been gained, in conversations with men already well known. The questions, as much as the answers, thus arose out of the historical context.

In order to illustrate these points in a running fashion, we will give parts or extracts of the interviews, followed by commentary. Then we will discuss the findings further, synthesizing them into a more general perspective. Mind and body are seen by these two men as in continuous interaction within the same plane of existence. The person's body is permanently made up of humors and substances, but its state at a given time is seen as a product of this interaction with the *noman*, and the *noman* itself is a product of the person's longer life history. The overall picture is therefore dynamic, not static. It is in this context that we need to understand the concept of the relational-individual that we have used in the writing of New Guinea ethnography (Strathern and Stewart 2000; Stewart and Strathern 2000).

## WÖMNDI'S EXPOSITION (APRIL 13, 1979)

### Extract 1

*Question*: As to the fact that people have different types of *noman*, please explain about this. When a child is born, does it have a *noman* or not? Does the *noman petem* (lie there) or not?

*Wömndi*: When children have only recently been born, at that time they do not have any *noman* lying there. No, they do not. They simply rest on the skin of their mother and breathe—they make *pung*, *pung*, *pung* sounds—they breathe. Their mother gives them the breast to drink, and so they continue until they are about two years old. Even slightly older children really do not have a *noman ingk* [true *noman*] either. Such children are attracted by anything that sways about or is colored red, that is all they look for as they go around. The presence of a true *noman* is something that comes a little later. But when the child is newly taken out of the mother, there is no *noman* at all there. That is something that holds for all children.

*Question*: Well, at that time is the *min* [soul] there or not?

*Wömndi*: No, at that time the *min* is also not there.

*Question*: Really?

*Wömndi*: Well, there is a situation where there is a *min* there. For example, when a child is about two years old and is still a small child being carried around by the mother, and it runs and stubs its toe or falls and cries out, that is a sign that it has a *min*. Or if anything hits them so that they are hurt and they cry out, then that shows that the *min* is surprised. . . . As for the time when the *min* will be properly there or the *noman* will be properly there [will lie straight], it is a little later when that happens, at about the age of five or six.

*Question*: How does the *min* come into people? How do people obtain a *min*?

*Wömndi*: Well, it happens that as they grow toward being adults, the breath [*muklnga*] inside them grows. The breath that was placed inside them grows. The *min* and *noman* grow. And the head [substance] comes to be straight inside them also.

*Commentary, Extract 1*

The relationship between the ***min*** (life force, spirit, soul) and ***noman*** (mind, will, intention) in Melpa thinking is complex. From one point of view a person's ***min*** comes from the ancestors and survives death to become a ghost (***kor***). In this view the ***min*** may be seen as implanted in the fetus before its birth and as evidenced by the kicking of the child while it is still in the womb. In Wömndi's formulation the ***min*** is also something that develops in the child over time, but only after its birth; and it grows alongside the growth of the ***noman***. The capacities of ***noman*** are clearly linked to development and maturation. ***Noman*** has to do with understanding the world, with reacting to events, learning from them. Wömndi presents the ***min*** as also reactive to the world, a principle of sense awareness such as the "knowledge" to cry out and inform others that one is in pain. The ***min*** possesses awareness of itself, so that it is then capable of being surprised. ***Min***, like ***noman***, participates in consciousness.

The concept of "lying straight" that Wömndi introduces is crucial here. "Straight" denotes that which is accepted as proper, as effective, as correct. Socialization is supposed to inculcate what is "straight," ***kwun***. Anger (***popokl***) is not "straight," it is "athwart" (***peta***). Anger reflects something that is awry in social relations, that needs to be "put straight." As the ***min*** and ***noman*** grow, they are supposed to make the person "straight" in this sense.

Wömndi uses also the concepts of breath (***muklnga***) and head (***peng***) here. Because the ***noman*** was originally thought of as residing in the chest, not the head, and because breath is a constituent element of spirit or soul in Christian theology, it is possible that his formulations are affected by introduced ideas. Lutheran Christianity had been preached in Wömndi's Dei Council area since the 1950s, and he would have grown up having some acquaintance with it.

## Extract 2

*Question*: People say that when a person dies, the ***min*** goes out through the fontanelle. Is that right?

*Wömndi*: Yes, that is true. When people are going to die, that is when their breath finishes. When we are alive, our breath makes us strong and we are able to work or decide things. This strength the ***wi okla wuö-nt*** [the man up above—God] puts into us in our breath, and when he takes it out of us and we think of walking somewhere and going, we are unable to do so and we have no strength in our skin. It is the ***peng konya*** [substance inside the head] that goes around and around and operates properly, and when that has gone out, then the person is just skin. The skin is there but the breath has gone out of it—the breath goes out and eats its food. When it does not come back in and look after us [***röp iti***] in that way, that is when we say that we see the person is dying. As we are asleep, it leaves our body to eat and comes back from time to time, and it asks itself how the person is doing. It goes off and it comes back and has a look, and then it goes off on its own pathways . . . and it quickly comes back, and it goes inside our skin and the breath comes back inside our skin. Then we awake and work. But if it does not come back inside, and up there at the edge [i.e., at a distance from the person's body] it walks around, and it just comes and has a look at where its owner is, then the person's skin starts to become small—the body shrinks. And the eyes become shrunken inside their sockets and . . . the ribs stand out. It is because the breath walks around at the back of the house and at the edges of our settlement. It simply looks at us from afar with its eyes and it looks from the edges, but its owner's body becomes smaller and smaller.

That is one thing. But if it stays with us, if our breath stays with us, if the heart is with us and it looks after us, then all of our skin is good and we eat our food. Its grease helps our skin, and our skin is good.

*Question*: When people die, they used to say that the *min* goes down to Mötamb Tilip Pana. Do you know about that?

*Wönmdi*: That is true. When people think that they are going to die, their *min* goes to Mötamb. Is that true or not? I'm not sure. . . . There is no one who actually goes there and reports later that this is what they have seen. That is why it is a rumor. People say it—that is just what we think.

### *Commentary, Extract 2*

The influence of Christian ideas continues to show here. Wömndi says that it is God (and not the ancestors) who has put breath (*muklnga*) inside us. He also says that it is *peng konya* (head substance, brain) that keeps the person operating, and when this no longer carries out its functions, the person is just "skin" [*köng*]. The ideas of *köng* as "body" and *min* as "spirit" were reshaped by Christian evangelists to express an opposition between body and soul that is very different in Christian thought from pre-Christian Melpa thinking.

Wömndi continues to refer to the *min* as the equivalent of "breath" here. "Breath" in fact comes to be depicted as the *min* of people. It is spoken of as going out of the body in sleep, and dreams reflect its explorations. A vital point is that the *min* goes out in search of its food. Like the body, the *min* needs food to keep going. And without the *min* the person's body in turn begins to die, marked by shrinking of the skin. As Wömndi elaborates on this, it becomes clear that the *min* is behaving in a way that suggests it has a *noman* or mind/will of its own. It can look at the person and decide whether or not to return to the body, and if it stays away, the person dies. The *min* here is represented as something that is potentially wild (*rakra*). If the *min* returns to the person's heart and "looks after" the body, then the body is healthy as a result of its "grease" (*kopong*) derived from food, and correspondingly the skin is healthy. Here it is not the *noman* that is presented as crucial to health, although the *noman* in fact also is said to function in this way. Instead it is the *min* that is in focus. Clearly also the *min* is a separate entity from the person in a way that the person's own *noman* is not.

Wömndi also shows the influence of introduced ideas when he modifies the picture of what happens to the *min* at death. Originally, the *min* was said to go to Mötamb Tilip Pana, an immense flat plain to the north in the Jimi Valley, where the Jimi River flows toward the Lai River. Wömndi now qualifies this as hearsay or guessing. He has in mind the Christian version, which says that the soul goes to Heaven or Hell.

### Extract 3

*Question*: Does the *noman* come to be with a person because adult people teach their children and so they learn?

*Wömndi*: Look, a child's parents see if the child goes down into a dangerous place or into an area where there are pieces of rubbish, and if they go down there and they wander among them, and they look and look and they play around, then the parents say, "Hey, that is something bad, don't take hold of that", or "if you do that, you will fall down," or "Don't do that—come back here." That is what they say to them. So we, the parents, who must look after them, we must be very strong. . . . I do this and I do this and do this. It is on the palms of our two hands that they have to grow up, and the mothers have to give the breast to the child. We the parents have to watch over these children with our eyes, and we have to keep doing it and doing it and doing it. Eventually the children grow up, and that is when they have a *min* and a *noman*.

*Question*: When children are small, are they said to be wild things [*mel römi*]?

*Wömndi*: They do not say they are wild. When our children are very young, we say that they are *nana* [little].

*Question*: What are the things that you call wild things?

*Wömndi*: Well, the things that are wild things are those which are out there in the bush. Living things that are found around the banks of the rivers, such as the river spirits [*kor wakl*] and those sorts of things that are around in that kind of environment, are the things that we say are *römi*.

The things that we people look after and rear ourselves or give sweet potatoes to—those are the things that are not wild, but the things that are just out there in the bush and eat food aimlessly [*roltinga*] with no particular customs, that find their food out there in the bush. These things just think their own wild thoughts [*noman rakra*]. Those are the things that are wild, but the things that are not, are the things that we look after. . . . We plant sweet potato gardens and we plant sugarcane and we plant bananas and coffee, and we rear pigs and have children and we marry. . . . These are the sorts of things and actions that we say are our things.

*Question*: Are all these things *mbo*?

*Wömndi*: Yes, these things are *mbo*. These are the things that we look after. We make them by looking after them [*röp etepon etemon*]. These are the things that come up on our two hands, by our own work. These are the things that I am talking about. As for the things that are *römi*, these are the things that you see up in the high forest or down there by the banks of the rivers—up at the tops of mountains like the Mbukl mountain, up at Miti Ku. . . . These we say are *rakra*. These are things like the cassowary or wild pig.

*Question*: But in the various gardens that are planted, are there some things that are the same as those that grow up in the high forests?

*Wömndi*: Yes, things exist in the garden that are also found in the wild state out in the forest, and we say that the birds have eaten the sweet potatoes and gone into these places and defecated. . . . That is how these things grow there, and that is how they can grow up randomly in the bush. These sweet potatoes are called the potatoes of bird feces. . . . There are fruits that grow up in a wild state in the forest, and we say these are *mel römi* [wild things] and then we take them and bring them inside our own fence. . . . We make them grow with our own hands and they come up, and then we say they are our things—true things—things of people because we look after them.

*Question*: There is a ***koeka***—a thing wild in the bush—a vine like sweet potato, isn't there?

*Womndi*: Yes, we say that it is like a sweet potato, and we harvest and eat it. Another is ***oka kombukla***, which grows in swampy places.

Pigs have a ***noman***, and people brought them in from the wild and then domesticated them. We can take their wild equivalents and hope they will turn into the domestic ones. We can do this with cassowaries. We find the wild chicks and bring them home and look after them, and then they become amenable [***wamb-nga ik pitim***, "they listen to what people say"].

*Question*: What about dogs?

*Wömndi*: There is a type of wild dog. This type is called ***kararip***. It lives in the big forests.

*Question*: These things that are wild do not have a true ***noman***, but what about a ***min***?

*Wömndi*: No, they do not have a ***min*** either. They don't learn what people say. If we were to tell them, "Hey, why are you here? Get out!" they wouldn't take any notice.

*Question*: The things with ***noman*** are the things that are ***mbo***, is that right?

*Wömndi*: Things that are ***mbo*** or domesticated are the things that become the possessions of us people. We carry them around and they really have ***noman***. A pig does have a ***noman***, but it does not lie straight in it. It doesn't really have a proper mind. A dog has ***noman*** but it, too, is not really straight. These two have ***noman***, but it isn't really proper. They will steal from their owners—those who have looked after them—and they have incestuous habits—they will copulate with their own mothers. These were wild creatures in the past, and so they have no ***noman ingk*** [true mind] now.

*Commentary, Extract 3*

The next part of the discussion turns on the distinction between domesticated (***mbo***) and wild (***römi***) things. Children are not "wild," because from the start they are brought up by people. Wild things are those which belong in the first place to the bush, beyond the arena of gardens and houses. Some wild things can be brought into domestic areas and can partly acquire ***mbo*** characteristics. And domesticated plant forms can also be found in the wild because birds have transferred their seeds there. Pigs and dogs belong to the realm of the ***mbo***, but their ancestors were wild and so they still have a partly wild nature. Therefore, Wömndi says, they cannot have a "true" or "straight" ***noman***, and he instances practices of thieving and indiscriminate copulation by pigs and dogs to illustrate his point. With children it is different. They are not wild, but they have no knowledge or proper sensibility. They acquire a proper ***min*** and ***noman*** only when they grow up.

**Extract 4**

*Question*: What about people?

*Womndi*: Take, for example, a man and a woman—a married couple. Sometimes they have a ***noman*** that goes straight, and they behave well together and they make business together. Whatever things there are, they work together at them. Only a few people are like that; . . . many people are really difficult with each other. Men leave women sometimes. Sometimes money comes into the home and the husband may not share this with the wife, even though she did a great deal of work in order for the money to come into her husband's hands. The husband may say, "Oh, you want some of this money, do you?" The woman may do a lot of work, and then the man may take the money . . . and spend it on beer or prostitutes. When this sort of thing happens, people say they do not have a ***noman*** that is straight. But some men listen to their wives and they will say, "We worked together, and this money belongs to us together, and we will use the money wisely."

*Question*: In general, do people have single or multiple ***noman,*** and do they lie straight (***kwun***) or crooked?

*Wömndi*: [Named examples omitted]. Men do not go around with a single ***noman*** and women do not go around with a single ***noman***. For example, the thoughts that men have are like this, "Oh, you woman, I could leave you and then marry two or three other wives." This is one . . . kind of thoughts that men have. The work that is needed to raise a bride-price makes us have many kinds of ***noman*** because of the effort involved in it. And men do not think of staying and living with a single wife until they die. Only a few men whose ***noman*** "dies" [is satisfied] stay with one wife, and women's ***noman*** works in the same way. They think in the same way. Only a few women think "Let me stay with this man and look after his children." But some women think "Why should I? This man upsets me. This man makes me feel ***popokl***. You are just a man, so why do you behave as though you are God?" Only a few people have ***noman tenda*** [one mind]. Both men and women tend to have many different ***noman*** [***noman kukla-ko petem***].

## *Commentary, Extract 4*

In this forthrightly expressed and closely observed section, Wömndi points out a clear ideal for a married couple: that they should work together for mutual ends and that their *noman* should accordingly be one, united, "straight." Quickly he adds that only a few people attain this ideal. Both men and women have "other thoughts," that is, they think of marrying another partner or they are dissatisfied with their present partner. In a polygynous system where divorce is possible, there is a kind of shifting marriage market that distracts people and destroys their harmony. Wömndi also mentions that husbands sometimes deny wives a fair share of the money their work has helped to earn. His remarks interestingly anticipate a national debate regarding polygyny that became intense in Hagen in the late 1990s (Strathern and Stewart 2000). The reference to God again shows recent influence. Because in the past there was no such concept of a high God and because people were not accused of trying to be like the ancestors, the nearest equivalent in pre–Christian terms would be to say "you think you are a 'big man' [*wuö nuim*], but you are only an ordinary person." Being able to point out that someone is not God introduces a new axis of comparison, that "we are all just human."

## Extract 5

*Question*: Why do some children stay small and not grow properly?

*Wömndi*: When that happens, there is something at fault, ***klawa ti petem-ko*** [a mistake lies indeed]. Something is wrong on the side of the parents. . . . For example, men may go and have intercourse with the sisters of their wives. That is something wrong that can happen. Or the mother and father of the wife may come and ask for something. They may request a gift of a pig or money or something like that or a cassowary, and then if the father of the child does not give the item, the ***noman*** of the parents is bad . . . and because they are ***mema tenda*** [one blood] with the child, there is a problem. Suppose you have children. Its grandparents say, "we think your children will do all right when they grow up because of your grease." They say this and leave because their ***noman*** is bad, and then the "man up above" [God] feels bad and the affairs of the children go slowly. The growth of the children is slow. That is something that goes wrong. If the grandparents of the children feel bad with the father or mother, then the children grow older but they do not become big.

Also, people say of some children ***tipu kuk titim*** [a spirit took their flower]. These children also are small. This happens when the child wanders at the banks of a river or in swampland areas; not here at our place but down in the hot valley places like Tiki and out in the swamps of the Wahgi Valley area. People go around and visit their food gardens and do work there: the gardening work, planting and weeding and harvesting foods; and food crops grow well in these places. And they put their little children in netbags and they suspend them there, and they go off and a wild spirit comes and takes the child away. The spirits look at the child in the netbag and the mother is working and doesn't see this happening, and they take their own baby that is bad, which they carry around themselves, and they put it into the netbag and take the good child off. They take the true child and leave the bad wild child and the mother harvests food and does not see, and she thinks the child in the netbag is her own child.

She takes the food and everything back home, and this child isn't her real child. It is a wild thing. The mother gives it the breast as she did before, but it doesn't grow big; its legs and arms don't grow straight. Its thighs are not healthy, and people say that the child is behaving as though it is a wild spirit. They try to give it all sorts of food—sugarcane, for example—and do all sorts of things, but it just goes wrong. The mother is in great pain, and she walks around and around with the child. She feels sick because of this and wonders what will happen with the child. She still thinks that the child will grow up, but its eyes are crossed and its mouth sits badly and everything is upside down and wrong with it. She thinks "My child wasn't like that before, but now it is." The mother doesn't understand that this is a trick that the wild spirits have done, and she is completely confused.

Those of us who understand about this thing and are going to leave a child like that in a garden area, . . . will tell an older child to stand guard over it. We as the parents say, "Watch over your younger sibling and do not go far off from the place of the child." So we leave the child and go off. It is as though an older child were looking after a second child and saying "I must look after it." Some children don't know about this. A mother can consult experts who live near where the spirits are, and can take the spirit child back where it should be, and they put it back. But some mothers don't understand about these experts and they continue to look after the child.

*Question*: Is frequent intercourse necessary to produce a child, or is a single time enough?

*Wömndi*: With a young wife it is not enough to have intercourse just once. The husband and wife will do the work of this for a whole year. Now as to how a child starts in a woman's womb, which we call her apron, *nggil*, we say that some women's wombs are soft, while others have two things that stand up from inside their womb like two beans [*pangila pök ropa-mel tetem*], and so they will become pregnant quickly. Such a woman will get pregnant quickly, and after about five or six or eight months she bears the child.

*Question*: Does the man's semen [*kopong*] go in and make a package [*kum*] with the woman's blood [*mema*] and form a child?

*Wömndi*: Yes, yes. But if a woman's womb in which a child is conceived is not strong, then the couple will have intercourse for a year or two or three or more years, and bear a child only if God above takes pity on them and helps. In the past they used to say *nanga pukl wamb, nanga anda kuwa* [my kinfolk, my grandfather], why do I not get a child?

*Question*: As to *ndating* [male ability to produce a child], is it something to do with this business of getting children?

*Wömndi*: Yes, they speak of the origin of the *ndating*. It is the man's genitals that are referred to as *ndating*. They say that grease [*kopong*] is there.

*Question*: Where do you think this *kopong* comes from? Does it originate in the head or backbone?

*Wömndi*: It comes from the marrow of the back or spine. It is that which gives birth to children. The marrow or fluid comes out of the spine and goes into the penis. This marrow of the spine goes into the woman. It is the grease of the woman and man that join together, and a child is formed in that way. It is the man's *kopong* and his *mbukl tiköm* [spinal marrow] together that go into the woman and cause the child to be conceived.

*Question*: Where does *mbukl tiköm* come from? What is the material in the head?

*Wömndi*: Spinal fluid goes with the grease of the woman, and the grease of the female and the grease of the man join together there, and that is how they say that a child will come to be born.

*Question*: Where does the spinal fluid or marrow come from?

*Wömndi*: From the *peng konya*. The spinal fluid goes into the head, and there it joins with the *peng konya* substance inside the head. They think the substance in the head and spine make the grease of the man, and it goes with the woman and that makes a child.

*Question*: What about the *noman*? Is it in the head or the heart?

*Wömndi*: It is in the heart [*muntmong*] that words and actions are thought, and then these are carried up into the *peng konya* [the substance in the head], so whatever they are thinking to do, . . . they join it there in the head, and after that it is the substance in the head that carries out things and has the capacity to do things. And that is how they do their work and carry things along.

*Question*: Is that why they have the phrase *peng konya penditim wuö*—a person who has a large amount of substance in his head?

*Wömndi*: That is said of someone who has substance that goes "straight." There are two versions of this term. One is *konya*, and one is *koya*. *Koya* is central Melpa dialect.

The *peng konya* communicates down to the *noman*, and the *noman* and it go together. And people say "I want to go there or there." It is the *noman* that is outside of the heart, and it is the thing that makes judgments, but it is only with the aid of the *peng koya* that it goes straight. If the substance in the head is finished, then they say that some other thing has come and eaten up the substance in your head. When you think of words, it will be like a wind blowing and the words will be like the words of small children; . . . such people carry on and say all sorts of "other" [inappropriate] kinds of things. It is only when in a man's head the head substance is really there "straight," and is made to be there, that people speak properly. There are some men who speak powerfully, and whatever they say and do, it is the *peng konya* that speaks down to the *noman* and tells it to say this thing or that other thing. It goes from the *peng konya* to the *noman* and from the *noman* to the person to say the thing. It is only because the *peng konya* makes things . . . strong, and gives judgment to people and strengthens them, that they are able to do things in an effective manner.

*Question*: They speak of *muntmong* [heart] and they speak of the *noman*. These are two different words. Are these two things different? Are they the same?

*Wömndi*: These are different things. They speak of the heart as when there is a *mbo* [a stock] in the *noman,* some formed intention in the *noman,* and then the people feel a certain *noman* [thought] in their heart . . . and they say, "Let me do this or that." It is with this *noman* also that they think to do this or that. They say that they think of it with their heart, but it is up there in their *noman mbo,* their formed intention. They think it and then do it. Their *peng konya* is brought in to make a judgment about it. "Let me go and do this or that," they say. And it is the formed intention [*noman mbo*] and the heart that must come together in order for them to have a single word or make up their minds.

*Question*: What about *kitim* [stomach, intestines]?

*Wömndi*: There is nothing in there. Only hunger is there. When we are hungry and we want to do work, we are unable to complete the task. . . . We are like someone who is sick, and we just sit still and we bend our head.

*Question*: What about the liver [*kaemb*]? To feel liver for someone means to feel pity or sympathy, doesn't it?

*Wömndi*: Someone says "It does not go smooth [*romint*] with me, and I feel sympathy." If it isn't *romint,* then there is sympathy and it is something of the liver.

About the heart they say "My heart is in pain," so they say pain is felt in the heart and it is placed into the *noman,* and they say something. Suppose they have stolen something of yours or somebody has died or some relative has been killed, and they tell you. . . . Then you say, "I feel it first in my heart." That is where it starts. It first cuts them in the heart, and they say, "Oh, my mother, they have taken that thing of mine. Oh, oh. It cuts me in the heart." It has made this *pukl* [beginning, root]; they feel bad in their heart, and then they also say they feel bad in their *noman*. If someone says, "I think I'll give you something" or they say, "Let's go and eat something," when this happens, a good feeling comes into the heart. Then they think "Oh, I'll do that." They think this first in their *noman,* but it begins in the heart. If they say there is something they forgot when going off to do a particular task, then they say, "Oh, I had better go and get that thing." This happens because at first we think straight inside the head.

*Question*: There is an expression in which they say that the *noman* lies across something or is not straight. What is that?

*Wömndi*: That refers to the ***noman*** in a person, to someone who takes things slowly. If someone says, "I've come and we should do this or that," the person to whom he speaks asks, "What is this, and why should we do this?" Such people ask these questions slowly and calmly, and that kind of person is one who has a straight ***noman***. But if someone comes and says "Let's do this," and the person gets aggressive, we say that the person has a crooked ***noman***, for he replies quickly and aggressively. His ***noman peta ronom*** [lies across], and the ***noman*** is not straight.

*Question*: What about rates of growth between boys and girls?

*Wömndi*: A child will grow quickly if treated well and fed. They sometimes say a girl is born first because she kept the boy down. Some children want to come out first and keep the others down inside. If a couple has many sons, then some are slow to grow.

*Question*: What about twins? Did they ever kill one?

*Wömndi*: [No, but] they would sometimes say, "Let's divide them so that they will grow well." One goes to the father's and one to the mother's people. So they share twins and there are enough people to look after each of them, and they thrive. The parents would find this hard to do by themselves. The mother's people get one so they should feel good in their ***noman***. They say one is for the ***kopong*** (grease) of the father and one is for the ***kopong*** of the mother. . . .

*Question*: If they are born at the same time, do they have the same ***noman*** or different ones?

*Wömndi*: No, they have different ***noman*** [***noman elpa elpa***].

*Question*: Really?

*Wömdi*: Yes, they may be twins, but still their ***noman*** develops differently and separately, as I have said.

*Question*: All right, on another topic, why is it that some boys grow up to be "big men" and others do not? Does God put the ***noman*** in people, or how does it come into being?

*Wömndi*: It is by the ***noman*** that everybody acts strongly. It is the head substance ***peng konya*** that takes this strength from the ***noman***. Some people have a foolish ***noman*** and there is wind that blows in the substance of their heads, while others take on the customs and powers of the fathers and their ***noman*** is cool [***ndi-ndi***] and there is a kind of strength that is there. As for the sons of a particular father, there is perhaps one who takes the customs and strength of the father, and he is the one who works strongly and takes onto himself the strong words of a "big man" [***wuö nuim***]. Some men do this. These kinds of men have pigs available for exchanges, and they say to themselves that they want to do the sort of things that a person who is ***nuim*** does. Others do not do that, and thus they do not become ***nuim***.

*Question*: The leader Ndamba has no single son that has taken on his power. Do you think he divided up his capacities?

*Wömndi*: Perhaps he did, giving work capacity to one and his ***noman*** for generosity and politeness to the other. But Ndamba's true ***noman*** [***noman mendepukl***] has not gone to any single man [i.e., no son has succeeded to all his capacities].

*Question*: Sometimes a father and a mother both have a strong ***noman*** but their child becomes foolish [***wulya***].

*Wömndi*: Yes, this does happen, too.

*Question*: Well, I see that your little son is sleeping, so it's time for you to stop and take him home now, isn't it?

*Wömndi*: Yes, I'll take him home.

*Commentary, Extract 5*

Growth is a physical process, but it takes place in a moral context. In fact, the health of a child directly reflects the moral state of its parents and is therefore a function of their ***noman***. Or, rather, it is a function of the exchange relations and transmissions of substance that the parents engage in. The mother's parents are particularly influential here, as the givers of a wife who brings her fertility and labor into the marriage. Wömndi ties all this in with the Christian God, suggesting that if the grandparents are annoyed, God feels bad on their behalf. The upshot is that the child will not grow properly.

Wömndi then mentions a separate phenomenon, the replacement of true children with the children of wild spirits. In these cases the parents try in vain to make the spirit child grow, but it just "comes out wrong." Wömndi does not mention if there is a way to get the real human child back. His example is the exception which proves the rule that children are not "wild." Only "wild spirit" children are wild, and when they are transposed out of their wild order, this is morally wrong and they do not grow well. True children are ***mbo***, they belong properly to the stock of their parents.

Wömndi goes on to discuss the conditions of conception of children. He mentions the influence of God once more (slotting God in where the ancestors had been).

In a continuous sweep, he moves on to his picture of male "grease" in the body and how this is linked to the ***noman*** or mind. His discussion comes back to a point that first appears in Extract 2, the role of the substance in the head, ***peng konya***. Head substance, spinal fluid, and semen are all one thing, so the reservoir of male conception material is what is in the head. Wömndi does not seem to expound on how this is supposed to work for women, but vaginal fluid, breast milk, and grease are all categorized into a single fluid system that also includes spinal fluid in women. We come full circle in our picture of body and mind when we see that Wömndi links head substance and ***noman***. Appropriate and potent action requires the cooperation of both of these elements, he says. Thus head substance is both a vital fluid with procreative power and an indispensable ally of the mind or ***noman*** in his scheme.

What we would call the mental and the physical are a single interactive domain, in which the heart also plays its part as an originator of feelings. Such a scheme entirely cross-cuts divisions into mind and body or thought and emotions, but it does indicate the importance given to judgment and assessment, signaled by the head substance, ***peng konya***. Also, the close connection between head substance, ***noman***, and heart indicates a reason why "the body" becomes a prime site or register of moral interrelationships. In Wömndi's scheme it is as though the ***noman*** provides the verbal articulation for certain feelings that originate in the heart, but both feelings and intentions also pass through the head substance. It is apparent from this scheme that because the *noman* and the head substance together produce the words that announce intentions, words are on the same bodily plane as the agencies that produce them. Once again, there is no clear categorical difference between words and substances, and this is an important clue to ideas of how magical spells, along with material substances, are thought to bring about results.

As noted earlier, this linkage of head substance with *noman* may be a recent one, but we cannot be sure of this point. It is well established and logically presented by Wömndi, which argues for the supposition that he drew on an existing stock of images readily expressed in the Melpa language (from which these interviews are translated). Wömndi clearly privileges head substance, *noman*, and heart together as important sites of thought and emotion. The stomach and intestines, by comparison, are for him simply the seat of hunger, although the liver is the seat of sympathy. A bodily image is used to express this. If the liver remains "smooth," sympathy is not felt in it. Presumably, if the person thinks the liver has a rough surface, then this indicates that it is disturbed and active in sympathy. The rough surface is like a bump or *mong*, which also indicates "trouble," a problem, something calling for a compensation payment.

Wömndi finally enters into another experiential realm: the differences between people. Twins may be born at the same time, but this doesn't make them have the same *noman*, because they develop differently. A "big man" cannot ensure that any of his children will succeed to his capacities. These points are grounded in the observational world of experience. There is no ideology or dogma that *noman* can be shared or inherited in a particular way. This underlines the fact that the concept of the *noman* provides a way of discussing processes in the world that are tied to perceived personal qualities and capacities. The interview with Ongka that follows considers some of these same issues.

## ONGKA'S EXPOSITION (APRIL 20, 1979)

*Ongka*: As for us dark-skinned people, I will talk about how different persons, important people and others, have different minds. I, the son of Moka, will discuss this. [At this stage Ongka had begun calling himself the son of Moka, referring to his prominence in *moka* exchange. His actual father was Kaepa]. We people of Hagen here can provide various examples. Take the case of a big man who may marry many wives—say he has four wives or five wives—he marries many wives and is thus an important big man. Really important men may marry ten wives or eight wives, and among these there will be one woman who behaves in a particular way. I will speak now about the minds of women. Later I will speak about the minds of men.

So, all the wives are there and this one takes it into her head to think the following thought: "I want to get this big man for myself. I want to stop him from keeping on marrying other women." So she makes up her mind about this and she decides to tell a lie. And so she says, "I have just eaten a leg of pork that he [the husband] gave me. That man is abandoning some of you other wives, and he brought a big piece of pork into my sweet potato garden secretly and gave it to me. He brought it to me at the edge of my garden, and I ate it." So she tells a lie in this way, and she gives evidence of this by taking grease from the gourd where she stores her own pig grease. She shakes the gourd and puts her finger into it, and with that she smears the grease on her face and her mouth and over herself. She says, "I ate this pork, and you can see the grease of it on my face."

So . . . she lies in this way and thinks that she will . . . get rid of the other wives. So she thinks this and says this, and one of the other wives says, "Ah, we all came equally to this man, so now he is turning you into an important woman [amb nuim], is he? He is turning you into something like his sister, is he? He is pushing me out, is he? Who was the person that I saw when I came here?" And then the wife who has been lied to takes a stick and hits the one who lied, and they fight each other. The husband comes along and asks why the two are fighting, and he says they are behaving in a *wölik* [jealous] manner. "What is this about?" The husband hits the woman with a stick—the one who started the fight. The woman says, "What! I heard something that made me angry. Now you are hitting me—I am dying of *popokl* [anger] about this." She takes her netbag and her flasks of grease and her large pig. She puts the rope on the pig and she runs away with it, saying she is going to go back to her own people.

So we the other men come along and start asking her what happened. Nowadays we make courts, but at that time we did not make courts, we just spoke in our own way and said, "Let's sort this out." And then we would shake all the talk out and we would see and say, "Ah, so this is the talk." A man asks, "What did you do?" and one of the wives says, "I saw that that woman had eaten a pig leg, and so I hit her." And then the husband says, "Well, I didn't take any leg of pork and give it to that woman. Who . . . gave it to her? What have you done?" The other woman says that this woman is lying, and the first woman says, "Me, lying? I saw the grease that you had on your skin—you showed it to me. I saw it." Well, eventually, they discover who actually lied, and they say, "You are a woman who goes around and makes many lies. You got into trouble, and we can see that you are going to kill your husband by sorcery."

Before, we didn't take people to court—nowadays we would take the woman to court. But we gave trouble to her. We said, "You are a woman who says bad words, you cut your words [*ketepa ropa*], you lie and "grease" others." Of a woman like this people say, "Let us not speak with her—she lies." When that sort of woman comes, we look at her and feel revulsion. She thinks again then in her *noman* and regrets what she did [*na petep nimb öndönt*]: "I did wrong and went around saying these things"; "I was wrong to have done this—I got into trouble." Then she feels ashamed and afterward she does not say things like that. This is an example of the . . . sorts of thoughts that a woman might have and that lead her to tell lies. One kind of woman does that.

Now let me tell you something about the minds of men. There is something that people do when they want to "break something off" from another person and get it. People have different minds about this. A man who has *noman kopa* [a true mind] truly gives his pig to the other person, and he truly takes things back if shells or pigs are given. He truly gives money and takes money back. But there is another kind of man who walks around and is eaten up by rubbish, and he . . . says rubbishness eats him. "I feel this, and I also do not work or rear pigs. What will I do? I will go and say that I have left a big pig at home and that I have a lot of money and a large cassowary, and I will ask someone to give me something quickly, quickly, at once [*pöt pöt ngui*]." And they give it and he takes hold of it. He holds it and takes it home and pays off old debts, or he takes it home and just eats it. And then he goes off somewhere else, and when someone comes and asks a return for it, he says, "I really don't have anything." And so his partner says, "You greased me and got that from me." Then he replies, " What you say I said, I did not say. I did not go to your house and ask you to give something to me. You just came and gave it for nothing. You gave it freely. I haven't got anything." He keeps saying things like that.

As for people, their bodies, eyes, and legs may look alike, but in their *noman* they are very different, and because people may have very different thoughts in their *noman*, they tell lies. There are men like that, but there is the kind of man who has another kind of thought and says. "If I were to do that, I would get into trouble and there would be people looking at me. I will die of shame, I think, and so I don't think I'm going to do that." Therefore, he truly gives something and takes something back, and truly does his work and truly eats his food. They say, "That is a person who goes strongly [*rondokl porom*] and works correctly, he has a true *noman* that lies inside him [*noman kopa petem*], he does not tell lies or grease people." And they say, "He speaks truly, so let us truly give something to him, and then we will truly get back something from him."

Another example has to do with people who think they will let someone look after something for them. If a man has a true *noman* and we give something to him, he looks after it well. Another man may say about your thing, "I'm looking after it well," but he will actually take it off somewhere and he will steal it. . . . Then he will come and say someone else stole it—he will lie and say that he doesn't know who took it. He'll be lying. He will cut down a cordyline and he will say, "Let us burn the *mi* [sacred totemic object on which oaths are made] and see what happens." He will lie, and they do it and nothing happens. . . . They say, "He deceived us and hid, he took something and ate it. He has got into trouble with us."

So there are people who speak truthfully and there is the kind of man who tells lies, and there is the kind of woman who tells other women lies and then there are women who say, "If I did that I would get into trouble." And so instead of deceiving others, such a woman truly rears pigs and gives things away and she works in the gardens. She thinks that if her husband walks around and comes home he will be hungry, and she thinks that the pigs will go hungry and her children will go hungry . . . and so she thinks about that and acts accordingly.

There is another kind of person who sees a man with a woman, and if she is hungry and asks for some food or asks for a smoke and says, "Where are you on your way to?"—or maybe smiles while speaking—the man sees this and he says, "Those people are up to something, some trouble is happening between them and they are arranging to do something." Some people say that sort of thing. Perhaps the words were innocent, but the viewer goes off and says, "I saw that." . . . Then the relatives of the woman come and beat her, and she says, "I didn't do anything! Why do you say this? Who told you this?" Then that person says "I was there, and you two came and said something, and I saw you." The other replies, "I was simply chatting with the person, why are you lying?" This is a kind of lying [*ik ketepa*, "cutting talk"]. When this kind of talk comes, they say it will "eat the ground," meaning that there is trouble and people fight. They say "Someone made this talk, and a trouble [*mong*, "a lump"] has arisen here. There is some kind of debt or a broken-off piece [*pund*] out of place now" [i.e., compensation will have to be paid for the trouble caused by the talk].

If we find out that someone has spread a false rumor of that kind [making *ketepa*], then the relatives of the person who has said this come and say, "So there has been a disagreement and talk has gone back and forth. Stay quiet now. I am going to say how I see it. As in the old story, when someone says they saw something in another place, they tell it untruthfully. Afterward you should experience shame and not repeat it again."

There is a saying: I see the tip of your nose, your lips, your eyes. I see that you are speaking in that way. The person who did that in the old days spoke a strong word, and after that there is someone who does not usually say anything but suffers pain, but you are the one who spoke about this. You said it for no reason, and that person has felt pain on the side of their skin and in their ***noman*** . . . that is because you told a lie about them and by your words you put that shame onto their skin . . . it is just because you told that lie about them, . . . and I advise you to stop doing that now." That is what they say to put a stop to this way of behaving.

Nowadays, if we take people to court, we take money from them or put them in jail, and afterward they repent or regret what they have done. They say to themselves, "Let's not do that to anybody again." . . . Before, we would say about a woman who did that, that she was a thief. Now we speak of rascals. Before, we spoke of those who stole and ate and went around. Someone who behaves like a spirit who eats and goes around, that is how they are. Now we see the real character of what they do.

For example, they would go to the group of the person and ask about the matter. There are people who lie in this way, but there are men who are very strong in finding this out. They look and listen, and they have power to find this out. They look at their lips and the tip of their nose and they say, "I can clearly see that you are lying."

*Question*: About people having different kinds of ***noman***, does a daughter take the ***noman*** of her mother or her father, and does a son take the ***noman***, of his mother or father?

*Ongka*: One son may take the true ***noman*** of his father. If the father has a true ***noman***, the mother may have a ***noman*** that is foolish. Men marry women from other groups. If the father has a strong ***noman***, the ***noman*** of the mother may be a foolish one from another group . . . Sometimes, however, this is a true ***noman***. Now you see this also on people's skin. Some people have a good skin and others have a bad skin. As there are different skins, also there are different ***noman***. When a couple have sexual intercourse, the grease that they have is mixed. There might be some bad grease that would mix with good grease. This grease alters things, it is an ***mbo***. It makes a formed packet. The father may have a true ***noman***, but the son may become foolish. If that happens, it may be that the grease of the mother caused that. Or it can happen the other way around, that the mother has a good ***noman*** and the father has a foolish ***noman***, and they mix. It would have been a good thing if the parents had come from one place, that would have been good. There are people of different groups, and we do not marry inside our own group. We bring women back from different groups. The grease from these groups is different, and it mixes to produce the child. The source of everything lies in the mixing of grease.

*Question*: Do young children have ***noman*** or not?

*Ongka*: Young children do not understand many things, and must be taught. After the upper and lower teeth have come and words come up into the head and they begin to make a noise in the fontanelle, then a child starts to realize things more clearly. Children begin to realize that things can hurt them, or they are hungry and they cry. The ***noman*** is not strong at this point. When a child grows up, then its ***noman*** comes up straight. Until then, we see the pulse on the child's head. When it stops, then we say the ***noman*** is truly there. When it pulsates, we say that wind goes into it. The head lies open and wind blows in it, and it doesn't have a true ***noman***.

*Question*: Does the ***noman*** come by itself, or do the older people teach the child and then the ***noman*** comes?

*Ongka*: It is just there by itself. No one teaches it. It doesn't work until it is shown things. The ***noman*** is there. It goes around and is foolish, and parents see that. And if it is a daughter, a mother shows a netbag and says, "You should dig up sweet potato and put it in the netbag." The mother shows the daughter what a digging stick is and how to fill a netbag and how to take the food home. "You come with me and do as I do. I will take greens also, and you can use your little netbag and I'll use my big netbag," she says. If it is a boy, the father makes a small axe for his son, or if it is an arrow that he is making, he makes a small one for his son. If they are going out to fight, he will say, "You take the small one and I will take the large one." That is what they say. He gives the son a small axe and says, "I'm going to cut down a tree here. You go and cut a small one there by my side. I'll show you how to do it, and when you see that, you take your axe and you cut one like that. You must watch to see that I make downstrokes and some sidestrokes in cutting." Different cuts are made with the axe, and he shows the son how to do it and the son continues. And when the man is old, the son takes a large axe and a large bow and carries on like that. A daughter continues, too, and when she becomes big, her breasts appear. At this time she says to herself, "Let me make a big netbag in the way my mother showed me and let me make a big digging stick," and thus she is able to carry on by herself.

That is how they show everything that has to be done. They do not show any ***noman***. The ***noman*** is there. The child takes on understanding as things are shown to it. They give a measure to it. If a woman has a daughter, she puts the measure on all things for the daughter, and if there is a son, then the father puts the measure on all things for him. And that is how things work out.

*Question*: When children are small, do they have a ***noman***? Are children wild things? Do they say that?

*Ongka*: They say that a little child is a thing that is foolish. It is foolish and does not think thoughts.

*Question*: Then they do not say that it is wild?

*Ongka*: They do not say that it is wild.

*Question*: What are the things that are wild? Are they things that are in the forest?

*Ongka*: Those are the wild things. Like wild snakes, marsupials, and birds. As for people, who are ***mbo*** [planted], they do not say that they are wild. Of the things that people plant, they are like the siblings of the things that are wild. For example, among types of sweet potato there are vines that are wild and different. Also, bananas vary—some are wild and some are planted. Also sugarcane and taro, the ones we eat are the ones we take care of. These wild things exist and are the counterparts of domesticated things. The ***noman*** is also in domesticated dogs and pigs. They have some ***noman***. Marsupials also can be kept like dogs and pigs, and can be domesticated by being fed the foods that are given to them.

*Question*: Some say that above there is a single ***noman*** and below there are many—what does this refer to?

*Ongka*: Above there is one ***noman*** that strikes the ***noman*** that is below and makes it go ***nung nung*** [a noise], it makes ***ngu*** [another noise]. The person says, "I want to say this thing, but the ***noman*** up on top does this to the ***noman*** below. It makes it ***nung nung***, and thus I am not sure what I should do." . . . With one *noman* we want to do one thing, but then another *noman* or thought comes and it says to the one below, "I want to do something else." Now there are two thoughts there, and the *noman* is divided. The *noman* up above is striking the one below and making it go *nung nung*. Should I do this or that? We become confused, and the *noman* above strikes the *noman* below. We see that, and things go wrong.

*Question*: Are many thoughts sometimes above and only one below?

*Ongka*: Yes, there is only one below, but if the *noman* on top says to do one thing and the thought below disagrees, then the *noman* on top strikes the one below and makes *nung nung*. Above there are many thoughts, and disagreements occur. Plans go wrong when this happens.

*Question*: What about the expression that the *noman* lies crosswise?

*Ongka*: That is used for people who are aggressive. They use aggressive words and they do not think down into themselves before speaking. They do not speak down here. They speak quickly and push their nose ridges forward, and they run out and take things upward and use a stick and hit people, who say, "Hey, I haven't had a chance to explain what I'm talking about, and you are getting into a fight straightaway. I see you are someone whose *noman* lies athwart." The one who has a *noman* that lies straight, that person decides not to fight immediately. "Let me listen and understand properly what this talk is about, and when I have understood it well and then I decide to fight—ok." That is a person who goes straight, who understands the talk of others properly. The person who has a *noman* that lies athwart only listens to a little piece of talk and has not understood it properly. . . . Then people say to him, "You go and hit people, your *noman* lies *peta* [crosswise]. That is why you do that." A person with bad thoughts who comes out and fights has a *noman peta*. The other type of person has a *noman* that lies straight.

*Question*: Does the *noman* lie near to the heart?

*Ongka*: Yes. When we have a thought, the heart sends it upward and it comes out and shows itself on the nose and mouth, on the face. And it comes out in our words.

## Commentary

Ongka's discussion parallels that of Wömndi in several respects. He illustrates the experiential point that people have different dispositions and ideas with a number of vivid vignettes of altercations between people that arise out of trickery, greed, and unscrupulous searches for self-advantage, all of which are indicators of personal character. These variations he attributes to the *noman*. The concept therefore is relied on for the explanation of people's habitual tendencies, but people can also learn to alter their *noman* through experience. The idea of the *noman* enables character to be seen as more fluid and less fixed than it would be if it were seen as governed ineluctably by genetics or by humoral dispositions not subject to alteration.

Ongka is very concerned with the problem of lying and deceit, which he sees as a common part of people's conduct. All of it indicates that the *noman* is not "true" or "straight" in a person. A true *noman* is the product of a good response to socialization. In a variant usage, he sees the *noman* of a child as being present from the time that the child speaks, but it has to be shaped and informed by experience. Ongka also notes that people's exteriors may be similar but their internal *noman* are different. At the same time he argues that insightful leaders are able to detect lying from people's bodily appearances—their nose tips and their mouths, for example.

Ongka develops a theory of the mixing of grease that functions as a partial explanation for the fact that children do not necessarily succeed to the *noman* of a parent, arguing that the "grease" of different groups is itself different and that the mixing of grease which occurs because of exogamous marriage brings complicated results. We see here the notion that groups are not just socially different but are thought of as having different sorts of humors constituting them. "The source of everything lies in the mixing of grease," he says. It is important to remember here that grease is linked to the *noman* through the idea of head substance that Wömndi expounded. Thus, a woman from another group may have very different head substance from a woman within the group. Ongka goes on to stress that children have to be taught everything, not because they are wild but because they are foolish (underdeveloped) and do not know anything until it is shown to them.

Finally, Ongka gives an exposition on the relationship between the upper and lower *noman*. It is a dynamic model. The lower *noman* may have a clear intention, but the upper *noman* hits it and makes it "ring" (*nung nung*), and it becomes nervous. These are expressions to convey the idea of uncertainty and of feelings that come up at different times, seemingly from below (i.e., they come into consciousness). The Hageners have another expression that ties in here: "The first *noman* is true," that is, the thought that first comes to us is genuine (perhaps given by the ancestors) and should be acted on. Later the *noman* from above may strike such a thought and prevent the action involved. Once more we see that the image of the *noman* is a way of talking about experiential life in which the whole person is involved. This in turn reinforces the reasons why we have called this chapter "Mind Substance."

## A COMPARATIVE NOTE

Hagen ideas of the *noman* are central to their social life and their views of the world at large. We have seen how they enter into questions of morality, socialization, social status, gender relations, and the definition of the person as a "body–mind" entity. Perhaps the exploration of comparable terms found in other parts of the Highlands would yield a similar set of ethnographic insights (see e.g., Biersack 1998 on Paiela concepts, such as *nembo*). Here we look at a comparison quite close to home for the Melpa speakers of Hagen, among the Maring to their north. The Maring people speak a language that belongs to the same overall language family as Melpa (the Hagen-Wahgi- Jimi-Chimbu family; Wurm 1964), and Maring populations are to be found in the Simbai Valley of Madang Province and on the southern side of the Bismarck Mountains in the Jimi Valley, belonging to Western Highlands Province, as do the Melpa speakers. Some Melpa speakers live not far south of these Maring groups (LiPuma 1988:14–17; Rappaport 1968:8–12). Rappaport suggests that ancestors of some Maring groups, including the Tsembaga of the Simbai Valley, whom he studied, "entered the general area that they presently occupy from the south" (1968:8–12). The Melpa, however, are not the closest to the Maring in language terms; this designation belongs to the Narak speakers southeast of the Maring in the Jimi Valley.

Ethnographers of the Maring refer to the importance among them of a concept that is linguistically almost identical with the Melpa term *noman*. This is *nomane*. Cognate expressions also are found in the Wahgi area east of Hagen (Blowers n.d.:362, on *numan*), among the Ku Waru people of the western Nebilyer Valley (Merlan and Rumsey 1991:226–228, on *numan*), and in the Kuman language area, the main language in Simbu (Chimbu) Province east of the Wahgi people (Nilles n.d.:175). Nilles translates the Kuman term *nomana* (with variants *noman*, *nomane*, *nomano*) as "opinion, feeling, belief, intellect, soul, insight, 'heart,' thought, custom" (n.d.:175), which suggests a range of meanings equivalent to the usages found among the Melpa and Maring. Blowers (n.d.:362) also cites a variety of expressions in the Mid-Wahgi language referring to emotional states into which the term *numan* enters, such as *numan ka paim yi*, "a man with good thoughts" (i.e., one who gives generously to others), which is the same as Ongka's reference to *noman ingk* in Melpa, "a true *noman*"; and Blowers gives as a general translation for *numan* "thought, mind, will."

Merlan and Rumsey (1991:227), discussing Ku Waru usage, point out that the concept of *numan* "provides the main and standard way in which people can and do talk about the 'real' reasons for their actions" (referring here to A. Strathern 1981:282), and they go on to say that "autonomous motivation is regarded as the most highly valued reason for action. Engagement of the *numan* renders achievement or accomplishment" (1991:227); that is, it marks out individual contributions to the flow of social life. They go on to refer to the unfathomability of other people's intentions, the efforts people make nonetheless to parse these at least retrospectively in order to constitute intelligible narratives of events, and the various ways in which nonverbal revelation of meanings and intentions takes place (p. 228). All of these observations apply equally to the Melpa speakers north of the Nebilyer Valley, where the Ku Waru live. Significantly, in one of their text notes, Merlan and Rumsey point out that the unverifiability of states of the *numan* "is limited by the fact that to some extent the body is the mirror of the *numan*, providing the only direct evidence of internal dispositions" (Merlan and Rumsey 1991:364, n.8).

It is this particular aspect of the concept that we have found to be clearly illuminated in the expositions of Wömndi and Ongka examined above. It is of the greatest importance to realize that for the Melpa the *noman* is in an internal communicative relationship with other aspects of the body, making the body as a whole "mindful" (Scheper-Hughes and Lock 1987; A. Strathern 1996).

The body/person is internally complex, and the *noman* expresses this notion of complex internal communication, manifesting itself in actions that become constitutive of remembered events and perceived dispositions of people. Out of this complexity there can emerge habitual patterns of action that are analogous to custom. As we have seen in the translations of the terms *nomane* and *nomano* among the Maring and Kuman speakers, the term "custom" actually appears, though such a translation does not quite fit any of the contexts we know for *noman* among the Melpa and Ku Waru.

The ethnographers of the Maring have also given translations of the term *nomane* that go beyond what we know of the Melpa *noman* in a further way. In describing how Maring male shamans communicated with the Female Spirit, the Smoke Woman, as discussed earlier, Rappaport speaks of the shaman's *nomane* as his "animated, immortal thought stuff" (1968:119). And in a later passage, commenting on the concept of *yu miñ rumbin*, "men's souls' cordylines," Rappaport states that "in contrast to the *nomane*, which is immortal, the *miñ* is lost at death" (1968:125). He goes on to give details about the *miñ* that exactly parallel the Melpa *min*, saying that if the *miñ* is frightened out of the body by being startled, or is driven out by sorcery or witchcraft, the person may die (compare Wömndi's remarks on this kind of topic). Rappaport continues: "The *miñ* is thought to walk abroad in dreams, and . . . a sudden awakening may not allow it to return to the body. The *miñ* may, in short, be regarded as mortal life stuff" (1968:125).

In his Maring glossary Edward LiPuma (1988:231) translates *min* as "life-force, bodily consciousness or awareness," and *nomane* as "soul; culture, custom." Expanding on the idea of *nomane*, he writes (p. 46) that "*nomane* . . . embraces the social sentience of an individual and practice itself, and speakers may use it to mean social essence, belief, custom, or culture." In the same passage LiPuma writes that the *min* is implanted in early stages of pregnancy, and says that males get their *min* from their fathers and females from their mothers (not an idea we know from Melpa). "*Min* is the life-force or spirit being which dwells in a person's body during their life (although it departs temporarily in dreaming)." Given the father-to-son transmission of the *min*, he adds, "The individual *min* of clansmen derives from a common source and thus is a salient point of clan identity" (p. 46).

LiPuma's formulations do not imply that *nomane* is necessarily "immortal," except in the sense of referring to customs or cultural forms that in principle transcend individual lives. Nor do his statements about *miñ* necessarily indicate that the *miñ* is "mortal life-stuff." Indeed, the notion of *yu miñ rumbim* may be taken to imply that the *miñ* of the living and of the dead are intermingled in the substance of the cordyline plants; and the identification of the *miñ* with the shadow soul that goes out in dreams and returns upon the dreamer's waking, suggests that the *miñ* actually survives the body and is detachable from it. In a later work Rappaport also translates *miñ* as "soul, life principle, or shadow," and says, in regard to the ritual of planting the sacred red cordylines, that "some informants say that they are actually injecting their *miñ* into the plants" (1999:76). He adds that they are in any case identifying themselves with their land, and that an immigrant who grasps the cordyline plants assimilates himself into the group, "possibly mingling his *miñ* with theirs, but at any rate joining them and, in effect, rerooting himself in the land" (1999:76). *Miñ*, therefore, clearly has collective and transcendent aspects, as does *nomane*, for the Maring, and therefore is not simply the mortal life stuff of an individual.

Resolution of translation issues of the sort we have explored here is not easy. We suggest, however, that the translation problems have to do with the imposed effort to see categories as simple opposites, in terms of the dimensions mortal/immortal and individual/collective. From the evidence, it can be suggested that *miñ* and *nomane*, for the Maring, may overlap in their meanings rather than being simple opposites. Both perhaps refer to complex aspects of the person as a "relational individual," (Stewart and Strathern 2000) and also to collective notions such as group ancestors or the sacred power a spirit such as Smoke Woman can confer on shamans who represent their communities. Another difficulty is posed by attempting to see in these terms an opposition between the body and mind/spirit. *Nomane* as "thought stuff" may nevertheless have a material or embodied aspect, as has *miñ*, when it is seen as a substance communicable to the sacred cordylines through a person's hands. And both *miñ* and *nomane* thus participate in an overall cosmos of flows of life force that certainly transcends the individual but also certainly includes the human body.

Overall, Maring ideas seem to stress the collective side of experience, hence the emergence of *nomane* as a term for custom or culture. In Hagen (among the Melpa) and in the Nebilyer Valley (among the Ku Waru, who appear to parallel Melpa ideas very closely) it is clear that *noman* tends strongly to refer to the decision-making capacities and powers of individual persons (always within the ambit of sociality that is coterminous with *noman*). Perhaps this is correlated in some fashion with the greater historical development in Hagen of competitive exchanges in the *moka* system, linked to the moral and political activities and choices of persons seen as autonomous and responsible agents, as Merlan and Rumsey have noted (1991:227). Other differences that we can note here are the variations in marriage practices. The Melpa leaders were more apt to have several (in some instances, many) wives, thus fueling the *moka* system, than the Maring. This also no doubt produced different perceptions of self and provided different outlets for the expression of agency for both women and men, thus perhaps defining *noman* in variant ways in the two groups. Also, as noted previously, the presence of missions in the Melpa area has impacted indigenous notions of self in ways that appear to differ from the experience of the Maring.

One of our main points here is that the body aptly becomes the marker of such a concept of personhood, and the states of the body communicate the states of the *noman*. To this context, then, belong a host of observations made by ethnographers regarding body, mind, action, event, and morality, observations which stress that it is not substances as such that are active; rather, substances such as poison, blood, semen, or breast milk become active as a result of people's intentions (e.g., Ballard 1998; O'Hanlon 1989). Michael O'Hanlon puts this point well when he notes that among the Komblo people of the Wahgi area, "individuals attribute considerable potency to what they perceive to be the true disposition [surely the *noman*] . . . towards themselves of those with whom they interact most intensively"(1989:54). Hence the importance of retrospective confession for these people (Strathern and Stewart 2000). Consistent with this viewpoint, "the Wahgi have highly developed notions related to the harboring or secret nurturing of grievances," sustained until revenge can be taken (O'Hanlon 1989:66). It follows that people's bodily states reflect those intentions, and their bodily substances, such as female blood, may therefore become the carriers of hostile (or helpful) action. The ghosts, who see such hidden intentions, can visit sickness on the bodies of those who harbor those intentions, and who act on them to betray and kill their own group members. As in Hagen, the body becomes the marker of the mind and of actions premeditated and carried out.

Further Wahgi ideas belong to this same context. Examples are the practice of making a pledge on the impatiens flower, which grows in marshy places, as a means of preserving the safety of a clansman in war—the plant's watery stems represent the flow of good blood in the clan (O'Hanlon 1989:84); the identification of the fertility of land with the "grease" (*kopong*, as in Melpa) of its owners (O'Hanlon 1989:42); and the idea that the smell of sexual fluids from intercourse, on the skin of warriors, makes them vulnerable to enemy war magic (O'Hanlon 1989:42). All of these notions indicate the intertwining of body, mind, locality, and action that goes to make up a cosmos of correspondences and influences. It is in this sense also that we reaffirm once more the point of talking about "mind substance," as we have done in the title of this chapter.

## REFERENCES

Ballard, Chris. 1998. The sun by night: Huli moral topography and myths of a time of darkness. In L. R. Goldman and C. Ballard, eds., *Fluid Ontologies*, eds., pp. 67–86. Westport, CT: Bergin and Garvey.

Biersack, Aletta. 1998. Sacrifice and regeneration among Ipilis: The view from Tipinini. In L. R. Goldman and C. Ballard, eds., *Fluid Ontologies*, pp. 43–66. Westport, CT: Bergin and Garvey.

Blowers, Bruce L. n.d. *Middle Wahgi Dictionary*. Kudjip, Papua New Guinea: Nazarene Mission.

Damasio, Antonio. 1999. *The Feeling of What Happens: Body and Emotion in the Making of Consciousness*. New York: Harcourt Brace.

LiPuma, Edward. 1988. *The Gift of Kinship: Structure and Practice in Maring Social Organization*. Cambridge: Cambridge University Press.

Merlan, Fancesca, and Alan Rumsey. 1991. *Ku Waru: Language and Segmentary Politics in the Western Nebilyer Valley, Papua New Guinea.* Cambridge: Cambridge University Press.

Nilles, Fr. John. n.d. Kuman–English dictionary. Typescript.

O'Hanlon, Michael. 1989. *Reading the Skin. Adornment, Display and Society among the Wahgi.* Bathurst, New South Wales: Crawford House Press.

Rappaport, Roy A. 1968. *Pigs for the Ancestors: Ritual in the Ecology of a New Guinea People.* New Haven, CT: Yale University Press.

Rappaport, Roy A. 1999. *Ritual and Religion in the Making of Humanity.* Cambridge: Cambridge University Press.

Scheper-Hugnes, Nancy, and Margaret Lock. 1987. The mindful body: A prolegomenon to future work in medical anthropology. *Medical Anthropology Quarterly* 1(1):6–41.

Stewart, Pamela J., and Andrew Strathern (eds.). 2000. *Identity Work: Constructing Pacific Lives.* Pittsburgh, PA: University of Pittsburgh Press.

Strathern, Andrew. 1981. *Noman*: Representations of identity in Mount Hagen. In M. Stuchlik, ed., *The Structure of Folk Models*, pp. 281–303. London: Academic Press.

Strathern, Andrew. 1996. *Body Thoughts.* Ann Arbor: University of Michigan Press.

Strathern, Andrew, and Pamela J. Stewart. 1998. Seeking personhood: Anthropological accounts and local concepts in Mount Hagen, Papua New Guinea. *Oceania* 68(3):170–188.

Strathern, Andrew, and Pamela J. Stewart. 1999a. *Collaborations and Conflicts: A Leader Through Time.* Fort Worth, TX: Harcourt Brace College Publishing.

Strathern, Andrew, and Pamela J. Stewart. 1999b. *Curing and Healing: Medical Anthropology in Global Perspective.* Durham, NC: Carolina Academic Press.

Strathern, Andrew, and Pamela J. Stewart. 2000. *Arrow Talk: Transaction, Transition, and Contradiction in New Guinea Highlands History.* Kent, Ohio: Kent State University Press.

Strathern, Marilyn. 1988. *The Gender of the Gift.* Berkeley: University of California Press.

Wurm, Stephen. 1964. Australian New Guinea Highlands languages and the distribution of their typological features. *American Anthropologist* 66(4):77–97.

# CHAPTER 8

# Conclusions: Mediating Opposites

*Pamela J. Stewart and Andrew Strathern*

The materials presented in this volume represent not only the ways people translate sensory signals sent between themselves but also the ways that the entire cosmos is seen to be involved in the flow of substances. For the Duna the "grease" of the dead person's body is believed to bring fertility to the soil and replenish it. Similar ideas are at the center of indigenous Hagen views of how the human body interacts with and is a part of the overall cosmic cycle of substances (the "grease cycle"). Duna people practiced rituals in the past in which pig's blood was given to the earth in order to restimulate its fertility; and a dance, known as *pilaku*, borrowed from the nearby Hewa people, had as one of its purposes to make the earth hot (*tindi rorowa*) in order to bring back human health and productive gardens.

In all of these examples and the plethora of similar instances in the ethnographic literature on New Guinea and elsewhere, we see that a number of common patterns appear among the intricate variations characteristic of each case. These patterns have formed the core of our topic, humors and substances, and can now be reaffirmed or summarized as follows (see also Chapter 1).

First, there is a set of ideas about the most significant substances in the human body, of which we can cite blood, grease, and water in particular as examples. Second, there is a concern with the flow and management of these and other substances, in terms of ideas of balance between hot and cold and wet and dry conditions. It is this concern that justifies our calling these thought-worlds examples of humoral systems of ideas. Third, these ideas in turn are intertwined with and contribute to the definition of complex social relations between persons, especially in terms of gender and power. Taken together, this ensemble of notions and practices adds up to a kind of moral economy of the cosmos, in which the human body features as a central component. On the one hand, the human body is a part of the cosmos. On the other hand, the body's agency becomes central to this cosmos and to changes in it.

Propositions of this kind can further be used to comment on issues that have emerged in analyses of concepts of embodiment, personhood, social experience, and historical change in contemporary anthropological writings that deal with both New Guinea and elsewhere in the world. We are not concerned here to isolate any propositions as uniquely particular to New Guinea. Rather, our overall concepts are intended to facilitate the inclusion of New Guinea materials in wider geographically distributed patterns that have been delineated under the rubric of humoral systems.

First, with regard to embodiment, it is in large part through expressions that have to do with the interactions of humors, substances, and organs in the body that ideas of the emotions are articulated. For the peoples in the areas we have discussed, then, the emotions have a clear physiological basis. There is no realm of the psychological separate from the body at large, and the body itself is a distributed site of emotions, capacities, and tendencies (see Chapter 7). At the same time, this site is seen as open to the influences of spirit powers in the cosmos, whether we see these as disembodied powers or as other forms of embodied power. The person is therefore the meeting place or arena of all these influences. Yet our study of Hagen ideas of the *noman* (mind) indicates clearly that this does not mean the person is passive or simply a register of spirit forces or of other human social influences. *Noman* signifies the active agency as well as the moral responsibility of the person. There is a kind of duality between the *noman* and the rest of the body, because the *noman* cannot be directly seen and it is thought of as having a controlling influence on action.

But this duality is not to be seen as isomorphic with the Cartesian division between the mind or soul and the body, in which the mind is seen as immaterial and the body as material. Hageners say that the idea of the *noman* is indeed a way of talking about action and experience, and is therefore an approximate way of discussing these matters. But when Wömndi and Ongka (see Chapter 7) discussed the interrelations between "mind and body," they explained how the *noman* is constantly in interaction with physical substances such as the head/spinal fluid and with organs such as the heart. This explains the intimate symbiosis of mind and body in Hagen thought. Their discussions are quite comparable to those of the medieval theologian St. Thomas Aquinas (1225–1274 C.E.), who in his *Summa Theologica* deals with the spiritual and corporeal substances of humans.

Aquinas first considers the proposition that the soul is a body, advancing arguments that this proposition is correct, then rejecting them on the grounds that the soul is the first principle of life and is therefore not the same as bodily life. On the other hand, Aquinas proposes that although the soul is not a body, it is in a sense a substance, that is, something subsistent. He concludes that "the human soul, which is called intellect or mind, is something incorporeal and [yet] subsistent" (Aquinas 1956:6). His formulation here is rather reminiscent of the Hageners' notion that the ***noman*** is quite real (subsistent), even though it cannot be seen as an organ, and that it interacts with parts of the body; however, they do not equate mind and soul as Aquinas (and, after him, Descartes) did. But the Hagen view of ***noman*** also makes "mind" more intimately interactive with corporeal substances such as the ***peng konya*** (head and spinal fluid) than Aquinas allows for in his scheme.

The idea that the human person is a part of the cosmos (which includes other persons as well as the total environment), but also has a special place within it, helps to mediate debates that have arisen in New Guinea ethnography on concepts of personhood. The relational aspect of the person is contained in the idea that the person is intimately bound up with the cosmos, and the individual aspect is contained in notions of personal boundaries, of stimulated and motivated flows of substances across these boundaries, and of intentional agency exercised in action that makes a difference in the cosmos: what Aristotle called ***proairesis*** "choice," or "that which is up to us" (***to ep' hēmin***) (Aristotle 1955: bk. 3, ch. 2:83).

Social experience therefore consists in the dialectical interplay between these two aspects, which are marked in discourse about appropriate or inappropriate flows of substances and exercises of influence. Major tropes are employed productively to create images of experience by way of which people express this dialectical interplay. In Duna, for example, notions of desire (***kã***) and consumption (***naya***) frame discussions about witchcraft. And the senses are brought into play in various ways. Desire is caused by seeing good food and by smelling it. In turn the divinatory stick that can find witches smells them out, too. Proper consumption and sharing express all that is seen as good in the flow of sociality (see also Eves 1998:39). Improper consumption, the taking of substance and sharing it with other witches, expresses all that is seen as bad: the balancing of norm against anti-norm, in S. F. Nadel's phrase (Nadel 1935).

The good smells sweet, the bad is rotten. In Pangia the term for anger, seen as bad, is the same as that for things which are rotten and stink, have a bad smell; it is thought to come up in a person's nose (see Chapter 4). The person's emotions, if seen as overweening or inappropriate, are sometimes imaged as arising not from inside the body but from outside it. In Hagen, inordinate desire, ***kum***, can be spoken of as existing in stones that can jump into a person's neck as the person drinks water after consuming pork. Grease, the same substance that revolves through the cosmos and helps to renew it, is also the object of ***kum***, which leads in turn to witchcraft and cannibalism. In these kinds of images, the trope of balance in social relations is given a bodily expression.

Issues having to do with cannibalism fit into our scheme here. We have not highlighted this theme, partly because it tends to be either overplayed or downplayed in anthropological writings, and partly because a collection of essays on it has recently been published (Goldman 1999; see also Brown and Tuzin 1983; Eves 1998:39–43; Sanday 1986; Breton 1999a, 1999b; Strathern 1984). The term "cannibalism" encompasses a range of actions that all include the basic feature that some aspect of the human body is consumed: this can include flesh, blood, the bodily fluids released from a cadaver, or the vital life force of the body (through witchcraft). It is also important to mention two aspects of cannibalism in the present context. First, where forms of cannibalism were practiced in the past, they must be seen as having varying purposes: for example, to punish a witch, as among the Etoro and Gebusi (Kelly 1993; Knauft 1985); to obtain ritual power from dead kin, as among the Bimin-Kuskusmin (Poole 1983); or to consume the bodies of enemies killed in fighting, as among the Bedamini (Knauft 1985:121, although the specific reference is to a killing carried out ostensibly as a contract killing of a sorcerer or witch on behalf of a Gebusi sponsor: the Bedamini killed a whole community, in fact, and took the bodies as their "pay"). From these examples it is not possible to say that cannibalism was simply one way to ensure the flow of substances and powers between people. When it formed a part of ritual complexes of action, however, we can certainly say that its purpose was indeed to transmit special powers in this way (e.g., Poole 1983).

The second aspect we wish to mention is that for many people of New Guinea, as elsewhere, the theme of cannibalism is set into a larger world of imaginings about what constitutes proper sociality and also expresses basic human psychological fears, examples of which can be found in folk tales from Europe and elsewhere (see the brothers Grimm's fairy tales, for example). In this regard, the question of whether cannibalism was or was not actually practiced (in one form or another) becomes relatively trivial. A good deal of anthropological writing has centered on this issue, following the work of William Arens (1979), who suggested that many reports of cannibalism are examples of colonial mythmaking about the "primitive others," rather than being true (Arens 1979). Arens's point was well taken at the time, but concentration on the narrow issue of whether people in fact ate others or not has tended to obliterate the significant point that the theme of cannibalism sometimes enters into people's definitions of what is civilized behavior, and therefore acts as an important mythico-ritual operator in their scheme of the world and its history (compare Sanday 1986:27–55). The theme is therefore emphatically not one that is simply the product of colonial inventions or fixations. This becomes abundantly clear when we hear from elderly people, who remember the time when the first non–New Guineans entered into their territory, that "we thought they might be going to eat us." Both the Duna and Hagen people make similar statements, thus demonstrating a preexisting knowledge of a category of "outsider" who was potentially cannibalistic.

The Duna people of Papua New Guinea provide an excellent illustration of clearly defined mythico-ritual notions surrounding cannibalism. In one of their group origin stories (*malu*), they tell of how a culture hero of a particular group, the Songwa, came upon a group of Poli people in Yeru, near the Strickland River, who were holding a funeral, mourning for a pig that had died. They were preparing to kill and cook two children (in some versions of the story, a young woman of marriageable age) to eat as the funeral sacrifice for the dead. The Songwa hero, Kepepa, instructs them that they have got their rituals the wrong way round. When a person dies, they should take pigs, sacrifice them, and cook them for a feast, rather than killing and cooking people for a pig's death. He persuades them to adopt his viewpoint by removing the dead pig's body from the funeral platform, butchering and steam-cooking it in an earth oven, sprinkling salt on the meat, and offering it to the people to taste. The taste of the salt (a valued trade good) persuades them to take this step to end cannibalism. Kepepa instructs them exactly what to do, and how to cook and distribute pork, taking a share of it for himself. He uses it as an enticement for a woman whom he meets in order to bring her as a bride for his younger brother, who subsequently raises the proper bride-price for her.

This narrative of appropriate culinary preparation and consumption versus inappropriate consumption fits broadly with the Duna views of the world—for example, that there previously existed giants (*auwape*) on the earth who ate humans, and humans had to kill all of them in order to establish themselves. The stories of these giants are kept alive in a genre of ballads called *pikono* (Strathern and Stewart 1997; Stewart and Strathern 2000). The performers sing these ballads at night in darkened meeting houses (traditionally in men's houses). The listeners are not supposed to look at the singer while he narrates his story, but are allowed to express, through excited verbal articulations, their appreciation for particularly engaging actions of the heroic characters. The cannibalistic giants that are said to have been killed are thought to be physically represented in the landscape, where large limestone outcroppings are identified as their ossified remains.

This theme also fits with the image of witchcraft, a form of negative cannibalistic society operating within the community. The witch is thought of as eating people's *tini*, or life force, taking it out of the proper cycle of life and using it to augment her (or his) own power and vitality. The witch, like the Poli ancestors in the origin story, can be appeased or "taught" by an offering of pork to desist from desiring human flesh, but this may not work if the witch's desire for human flesh is too great.

Likewise, pig's blood can be a surrogate for human blood in gifts to renew the earth, although one ritual, the *hambua hatya*, required the killing and distribution of the body parts of a virile man who had sired children (Stewart 1998; Strathern 1998). Pigs, close in substance to humans, become crucial instruments of both a noncannibalistic social order and the cosmic cycle of renewal and substance flow. They obviate the need for human sacrifice or cannibalism, and they help to maintain the cyclicity of renewal between humans and the earth, preventing the earth from "finishing." Interestingly, when the first non–New Guineans entered the Duna area, it was thought that the outsiders were going to kill all of the people's pigs (and they actually did kill and eat many of them), and thereby cause the ground to "finish."

Perhaps a similar thought of cosmic connection and pigs as human surrogates lies behind a rule established in another Duna ritual, the *yeke yokoni*, whose purpose was to divine who would become a *kango* or prominent man in the upcoming generation of males in a community. Men singled out in this ritual were expected to be given pigs by others, and they were enjoined to keep such a pig if it was female, and allow it to reproduce continually. They were told not to kill such a pig for a funeral sacrifice, although later they could kill it for some other purpose. This rule appears to echo the Songwa story (*malu*): although it is appropriate in general to kill pigs for funerals, certain female pigs that are a mark of a person's success in pig-breeding should be allowed to reproduce as people do, and should be preserved. Just as it is not appropriate to kill humans in funeral sacrifices, so in this instance it is not appropriate to kill the pig. This rule constitutes an extension of personhood from people to pigs.

Another intriguing aspect of this ritual was that it began with the killing of pigs, extraction of their lower intestines (which are carefully cleaned by women), and the insertion of sharp pieces of flint and bamboo (both prepared for the occasion by men) into the cleaned intestines. The men were then lined up, and each compressed a section of a long intestinal tube, containing the sharpened flint and bamboo pieces, that had been sewed together. The man or men who had been cut so deeply that their blood flowed liberally were deemed by the ritual expert at the event to be candidates to become leading and successful men, (*kango*), who would have many pigs and cowrie shell wealth. The ritual here required pig sacrifices as well as human blood that came from the manipulation of pig intestines, exemplifying again the close relationship between pigs and people and their bodily fluids.

The person and the body are repositories of social values. They are also intertwined with the environment and its complex changes. In a striking number of instances people perform rituals specifically in order to set a disturbed environment to rights. Their rituals have what we would call ecological aims. The starting point for the descriptions of these rituals tends always to be the human body and the condition of its skin as a marker of well-being or sickness: *skin i lus* "[our] skin was loose," people say in Tok Pisin, indicating a lack of subcutaneous body fat and the need to build it up again. Equally, they may start with remarks about the skins of pigs or the small size of sweet potatoes. Practical issues of the utmost day-to-day importance in their social experience are combined with large-scale attempts to tip the balance of the cosmos in the right direction again.

An example of these renewal rituals can be seen in the narrative, collected from a senior Duna man in the 1990s, of the *kira pulu* cult ritual, which was practiced in the past by his father.

**Kira Pulu**

The ritual was performed when there was a time of famine, when young boys and girls did not appear to be developing properly, when there was a scarcity of wild game (including birds and marsupials), or when the marsupials of the high forest were eating too many of the nuts from the pandanus trees. [These nuts are a rich source of protein and fat for the people, and the trees are individually "owned" by men who mark them as belonging to them and who collect cultivate the nuts when they are ripe]. It was thought that ancestral forces caused these unfortunate occurrences to take place, and the cult aimed to appease these spirits. The practice involved the "feeding" of fruit and pig substance to ancestral skulls that had been ritually marked by an expert and gathered together in a specially constructed house by the sons of the men whose skulls were being used in the ritual. The skulls were of men known as ***kira haiyeni.*** The men who had obtained the status of ***kira haiyeni*** had been involved twice during their lives in the cult. A ***kira haiyeni*** man was marked out as the possessor of special ritual powers and was able to preside over rituals other than the ***kira pulu.*** He was also allowed to eat cassowary meat and a special type of marsupial, called ***wi homake***, which was forbidden to women, children, and men who had not been involved twice in the ***kira pulu.*** The ***kira haiyeni*** was thereby marked for special ancestorhood. When he died, his wife had to observe care at the mourning ceremony, where his body was laid out and women surrounded it, singing laments [see Chapter 4] and wailing. The wife was told to sit at the head of her husband's body and not to pass across his head. His skull was subsequently used in the ***kira pulu*** ritual.

During the ritual the skulls of the ***kira haiyeni*** men were placed in the ritual house and arranged in a row. An expert, who stood in a relationship of cross-cousinhood (***apa***) to the celebrants, dripped the grease from sacrificed pig kidneys into the opened mouths of the skulls. ***Suku*** bananas were suspended over the skulls and allowed to decay over several months, dripping their juices into the opened mouths of the skulls. During this time the building was sealed, and strict observance of a set of taboos had to be maintained: young boys were told to keep themselves clean and not to hunt birds, cassowaries, wild pigs, or rats. After a period of time, when the expert looked into the house and saw that the bananas and pork had completely released their juices, he began counting the days by making a knot into a rope for each day that passed . There was a restriction on having sexual intercourse during this time. When day number sixteen came round, the expert told each participant in the ritual to go into the house and retrieve his father's skull and return it to the secondary burial site in the high limestone caves above the dwelling places.

Here we see the cycle of substance flow and renewal of the ground clearly detailed. The ancestral spirits and the physical remains of their bodies retained a close relationship with the living. But with the coming of the missionaries into the Duna area, the people were told to abandon these rituals.

The question of historical change is an important one. If the body is a prime locus of moral experience, and if historical changes alter that experience, then people's bodies, too, are seen to change. In Pangia, as an expectable correlate of the fact that cults of renewal and increase were suspended in response to missionary teachings in the 1960s, there developed a notion that the people's bodies were shrinking in size (Clark 1989). (It is not impossible that these notions were also affected by awareness of the generally larger size of the Australian government officers who patrolled the area). Among the Duna, this idea of shrinking size is linked to moral themes and notions of cyclical decline prior to renewal. Young people are said not to heed their parents and to engage prematurely in sexual intercourse, depleting their energies early on and stunting their growth. The concern of colonial authorities with measuring people and computing the weights and growth rates of babies in health clinics may also have fed into these indigenous cosmological concerns. In any case, these examples make it clear that the body is indeed an important marker of historical change.

Discussions on the body in anthropology have tended to oscillate between a stress on the body as a passive marker and the body as a locus of agency. Mary Douglas is usually cited as a proponent of the first viewpoint, although this does not do justice to the subtlety of her work because she distinguished clearly between different social environments and their effects on perception and experience (Douglas 1966). Thomas Csordas has taken up the opposite pole of emphasis in his own work (e.g., Csordas 1994), emphasizing embodied experience as the foundation of culture. Douglas spoke of the "social body" as constraining the perceptions of the "individual body," thus enshrining an opposition between society and the individual (Douglas 1970:68). However, if we start with a different set of propositions, such as we have employed here, this opposition is mediated. To say that the body is a part of the cosmos implies that it has its place in the cosmos and that the cosmos, in a sense, runs through it, as well as vice versa. To be a part of the cosmos, however, is also actively to experience life within it, and to experience change and stress that evoke active and energetic responses. Ritual action channels these responses, which are also made in everyday activities. We can therefore see that both active agency and the passive registering of events are part and parcel of the experiential world. The notion of humors and substances neatly captures this notion. It presents a picture both of physical substances, their accumulations and depletions, flows and blockages, and of the active temperaments of persons who experience, make images of, and attempt to bend to their own purposes the cosmos in which they perceive themselves to be living, as both made by it and making themselves in it.

The idea of the cosmos here is perhaps the most important analytical notion that we have introduced into the overall discussion. As we use it, the term refers to the overall life-world of relations between people and between people and their perceived living environment (compare Coppet and Itéanu 1995). It therefore includes both the realm of "society" or sociality and the domain of "nature," here seen as an integral part of social relations, just as these relations are seen as embedded within the environment (for some debates on issues involved here, see Ingold 1996). The idea of the cosmos is clearly a cultural idea, but it does not necessarily imply a bounded cultural or social unit as such, because different areas may participate in an overall interregional picture of a cosmos that encompasses them. This was the case in relations such as the Duna conceived of in their concept of "straightening the ground" (*rindi kiniya*), in which ritual ties were set up between themselves and the Huli via the image of ritual trackways (Stewart 1998). The cosmos may also be seen as flexibly extensible and as subject to historical change: we are not dealing with a notion of timeless order but of enduring interrelations between people in a life-world. Seeing a social person as a part of such a cosmos enables us to conceptualize persons both as the sites of wider relationships and as intentional agents, because their agency is part of a wider cycle of the reproduction of relations. Humors and substances, in turn, belong both to the cosmos and to the person. Their flows are seen as maintaining the cosmos and at the same time as dependent on human agency and choice. Both human life and the cosmos exist also in the flows of time—seasonal, biographical, and generational—so that all life is seen as in a flux of growth, decay, extinction, and renewal, and the reckoning of temporal processes implies points of change within this flux.

It is in a context of this kind that Duna ideas of "the ground finishing" find their interpretive place. Established flows of substance maintain and renew the cosmos. Equally, new and deleterious flows are seen as threatening that cosmos, which in any case had in the past to be maintained by elaborate rituals. The advent of new epidemic diseases, particularly AIDS, into a life-world of this kind introduces the threat of death and extinction into the context of reproduction itself. How people such as the Duna will react to and cope with this threat will depend greatly on their existing theories of humors and substances, as well as on the quality of introduced health care in their communities. At this point, we are looking at the conjunction of ethnography and issues of applied public health, which would require a separate treatment of its own. Such a discussion would certainly need to take into account the implications of the ethnographic patterns we have been exploring in this book.

## REFERENCES

Aquinas, Thomas. 1956. *Summa Theologica. Pt. 1, Questions on Man.* Trans. by Anton C. Pegis. Chicago: Great Books Foundation.

Arens, William. 1979. *The Man-Eating Myth.* New York: Oxford University Press.

Aristotle. 1955. *The Ethics of Aristotle.* Trans. by J.A.K. Thomson. Harmondsworth, UK: Penguin Books.

Breton, Stéphane. 1999a. Death and the ideology of compensation among the Wodani, Western Highlands of Irian Jaya. *Social Anthropology* 7(3): 297–326.

Breton, Stéphane. 1999b. Le spectacle des choses: Considérations mélanésiennes sur la personne. *L'Homme* 149:83–112.

Brown, Paula, and Donald F. Tuzin (eds.). 1983. *The Ethnography of Cannibalism.* Washington, DC: Society for Psychological Anthropology.

Clark, Jeffrey. 1989. The incredible shrinking men and male ideology and development in a Southern Highlands society. *Canberra Anthropology*

12(192):120–143. Spec. iss. titled *Culture and Development in Papua New Guinea*, ed. Chris Healey.

Coppet, Daniel de, and André Iteanu (eds.). 1995. *Cosmos and Society in Oceania.* Oxford: Berg.

Csordas, Thomas (ed.). 1994. *Embodiment and Experience: The Existential Ground of Culture and Self.* Cambridge: Cambridge University Press.

Douglas, Mary. 1970. *Natural Symbols: Explorations in Cosmology.* New York: Pantheon Books.

Douglas, Mary. 1966. *Purity and Danger: An Analysis of the Concepts of Pollution and Taboo.* London: Routledge and Kegan Paul.

Eves, Richard. 1998. *The Magical Body: Power, Fame and Meaning in a Melanesian Society.* Amsterdam: Harwood Academic Publishers.

Goldman, Laurence (ed.). 1999. *The Anthropology of Cannibalism.* Westport, CT: Bergin and Garvey.

Ingold, Tim (ed.) 1996. *Key Debates in Anthropology.* London and New York: Routledge.

Kelly, Raymond. 1993. *Constructing Inequality: The Fabrication of a Hierarchy of Virtue among the Etoro.* Ann Arbor: University of Michigan Press.

Knauft, Bruce M. 1985. *Good Company and Violence: Sorcery and Social Action in a Lowland New Guinea Society.* Berkeley: University of California Press.

Nadel, Siegfried F. 1935. Witchcraft and anti-witchcraft in Nupe society. *Africa* 8(4):423–447.

Poole, Fitz John Porter. 1983. Cannibals, tricksters and witches. Anthropophagic images among Bimin-Kuskusmin. In Paula Brown and Donald Tuzin, eds., *The Ethnography of Cannibalism*, pp 6–32. Washington, DC: Society for Psychological Anthropology.

Sanday, Peggy R. 1986. *Divine Hunger: Cannibalism as a Cultural System.* Cambridge: Cambridge University Press.

Stewart, Pamela. 1998. Ritual trackways and sacred paths of fertility. In Jelle Miedema, Cecilia Ode, and Rien Dam, eds., *Perspectives on the Bird's Head of Irian Jaya, Indonesia: Proceedings of the Conference, Leiden 13–17 October 1997*, pp. 275–289. Amsterdam and Atlanta: Rodopi.

Stewart, Pamela J., and Andrew Strathern. 2000. Naming places: Duna evocations of landscape in Papua New Guinea. *People and Culture in Oceania.* In press. Vol. 16:87–107.

Strathern, Andrew. 1984. Witchcraft, greed, cannibalism and death. In Maurice Bloch and Jonathan Parry, eds., *Death and the Regeneration of Life*, pp. 111–133. Cambridge: Cambridge University Press.

Strathern, Andrew. 1998. Sacrifice and sociality: A Duna ritual track. In Laurence Goldman and Chris Ballard, eds., *Fluid Ontologies*, pp. 31–42. Westport, CT: Bergin and Garvey.

Strathern, Andrew J., and Pamela J. Stewart. 1997. Ballads as popular performance art in Papua New Guinea and Scotland. Discussion Paper no. 2. James Cook University, Centre for Pacific Studies.

# Index

# About the Authors and Contributors

PAMELA J. STEWART is a Research Associate in the Department of Anthropology and the Department of Religious Studies at the University of Pittsburgh. She has also worked as a senior visiting fellow, International Institute for Asian Studies, Leiden University, Leiden, The Netherlands. Her main areas of interest are gender studies, political and religious change, and medical anthropology. She works with her husband and collaborator, Andrew Strathern, in the Duna, Hagen, and Pangia areas of Papua New Guinea. Her most recent coauthored books are *Curing and Healing: Medical Anthropology in Global Perspective* (1999) and *The Python's Back: Pathways of Comparison Between Indonesia and Melanesia* (2000). She and A. Strathern have coedited a special issue of the journal *Ethnohistory* [47(1), 2000], titled "Millennial Countdown in New Guinea."

ANDREW STRATHERN is Mellon Professor of Anthropology in the Department of Anthropology, University of Pittsburgh. His interests are in the fields of political and legal anthropology, medical anthropology, and historical change in general. His most recent books coauthored with his wife, Dr. Pamela J. Stewart, include *Collaborations and Conflicts: A Leader Through Time* (1999) and *Arrow Talk: Transaction, Transition, and Contradiction in New Guinea Highlands History* (2000). His research is currently conducted in Lowland Scotland as well as Papua New Guinea, in collaboration with Pamela J. Stewart (Strathern).

DIANNE VAN OOSTERHOUT, ISIR-Ph.D, Leiden University, conducted research in Inanwatan in 1995–1996 within the context of the ISIR-program. This NWO priority program aims to study the Bird's Head area of Irian Jaya and to integrate multidisciplinary knowledge.

IEN COURTENS, is a Research Associate, Centre for Pacific Studies, Department of Anthropology, University of Nijmegen, The Netherlands

www.ingramcontent.com/pod-product-compliance
Ingram Content Group UK Ltd.
Pitfield, Milton Keynes, MK11 3LW, UK
UKHW041636031026
15587UKWH00001B/325

9 780897 897624